An Introduction to Mechanics of Human Movement

by

James Watkins

Scottish School of Physical Education
Jordanhill College of Education, Glasgow, Scotland

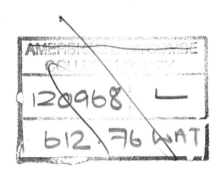

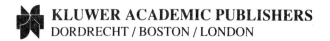

KLUWER ACADEMIC PUBLISHERS
DORDRECHT / BOSTON / LONDON

Distributors

---

for the United States and Canada: Kluwer Academic Publishers, PO Box 358, Accord Station, Hingham, MA 02018-0358, USA
for all other countries: Kluwer Academic Publishers Group, Distribution Center, PO Box 322, 3300 AH Dordrecht, The Netherlands

British Library Cataloguing in Publication Data

Watkins, James
    An introduction to human movement.
    1. Human locomotion
    I. Title
    612'.76   QP303

ISBN 0-85200-492-3 (hardback)
ISBN 0-85200-975-5 (paperback)

Published in the United Kingdom by Kluwer Academic Publishers, PO Box 55, Lancaster, UK.

Kluwer Academic Publishers BV incorporates the publishing programmes of D. Reidel, Martinus Nijhoff, Dr W. Junk and MTP Press.

Typeset by Blackpool Typesetting Services Ltd., Blackpool.
Printed and bound by Antony Rowe Ltd., Chippenham, UK.

Contents

Preface

Every person must organise his or her movement in relation to unique constraints of a developmental, morphological and mechanical nature. At any particular stage in the growth and development of the human body it is not possible to remove the developmental and morphological constraints but it may be possible by careful observation or other means to detect and thereby correct errors in movement due to unsound body mechanics. The correction of mechanical faults will result in more efficient and skilful movement. Every time a physical education teacher or sports coach attempts to improve the technique of an individual with regard to a particular movement, he or she is, in effect, trying to improve the mechanics of the individual's movement.

This book is designed primarily as a mechanics course text for undergraduate students of physical education and human movement. However, many of the sections in the book will be of interest to students of physiotherapy. In addition, I expect that the book will be of considerable interest to teachers of mechanics in schools since many of the concepts which make up the content of the book are the same as in any first course in mechanics.

The key to understanding mechanics is a thorough understanding of the concepts of force and Newton's laws of motion. Based on this premise, the content of the book is concerned largely with the development of an understanding of the effects of Newton's laws of motion with regard to linear and angular motion. All of the fundamental mechanical concepts are explained from first principles, and many examples from a range of physical activities are given in order to illustrate the practical application of the concepts. Unlike other texts in the field, no previous knowledge of mechanics is assumed as a prerequisite to the use of the book.

1

Introduction

1.1 Mechanics of Human Movement

Mechanics is the study of conditions under which objects move or stay at rest. The two states of 'at rest' and 'in motion' have led to a division of mechanics into two major areas, i.e.

(i) *Statics*, which deals largely with the conditions under which objects remain at rest.

(ii) *Dynamics*, which deals largely with the conditions under which objects move.

The term 'object' as used here and throughout the book refers to anything which has mass and occupies space, i.e. everything on earth, animate and inanimate. Mechanics of human movement is the study of the conditions under which the human body moves or stays at rest, and this book is concerned with the basic principles of statics and dynamics as they apply to human movement. There are two other areas of study within the mechanics of human movement which are not covered in this book but which should be noted. These are mechanics of materials and fluid mechanics. Mechanics of materials is concerned with the determination of the strength and deformation characteristics of the various tissues which make up the human body such as muscle, tendon and bone. Injury is simply the result of putting too much strain on the body tissues. Fluid mechanics is concerned with the study of the conditions which govern the movement of liquids and gases and the movement of objects through liquids and gases; for example, the study of the factors which affect the movement of blood in blood vessels and the movement of the human body through air and water.

Every object on earth is continuously acted upon by one or more forces. The concept of force is covered in detail in Section 2.5 but at this stage it is sufficient to realise that in order to move an object from rest or to speed up or slow down a moving object, it is necessary to apply an unbalanced force to the object. When the forces acting on the object balance each other, the object will be either at rest or moving in a straight line with constant speed. Therefore the motion of an object, i.e. the way in which it moves, depends upon the magnitude and direction of the forces acting on it. Force may be in the form of a push or a pull or some variation of these actions such as supporting, lifting, kicking and blowing. Statics deals with the determination of the forces acting on objects which are at rest or moving in a straight line with constant speed, i.e. statics is the study of objects under the action of balanced forces. Dynamics, on the other hand, is concerned with the study of objects under the action of unbalanced forces. There are two branches to dynamics, namely *kinematics* and *kinetics*. *Kinematics* deals with the description of the motion of objects. A kinematic analysis provides a precise spatio-temporal description of the movement of an object in terms of:

(a) How far the object moves (distance).
(b) How quickly it moves (speed).
(c) How consistently it moves (acceleration).

Kinetics deals with the determination of the forces acting on an object which are responsible for the movement of the object as described in kinematics.

It should be evident that a thorough understanding of the concept of force is essential in order to understand mechanics. The mechanics of human movement may be defined as:

> *The study of the internal and external forces acting on the human body and their effects on the movement of the body.*

1.2   Forms of Motion

There are two basic forms of motion, namely *linear* and *angular*. *Linear* motion, which is also referred to as *translation*, occurs when all parts of an object move the same distance in the same direction in the same time. For example, the movement of a car along a straight and level road would be an example of linear motion. Pure linear motion seldom occurs in human movement since in all types of self-propelled movement the orientation of the body parts to each other is continually changing and, therefore, all parts of the body do not move the same distance in the same direction in the same time. The human body may experience pure linear motion in such activities as skiing or skating provided that the supporting surface is perfectly even.

Angular motion, also referred to as *rotation*, occurs when an object or part of an object such as an arm or leg moves in a circle or part of a circle about a particular line called the axis of rotation, i.e. each part of the object moves through the same angle in the same direction in the same time. For example, a wheel undergoes angular motion when turning about its axle. Similarly the movements of the limbs of the human body about their respective joints are examples of angular motion. Most movements are combinations of the two basic forms of motion. For example, in walking, running and swimming, the movement of the body as a whole may be linear; however, this is achieved by angular motion of the arms and legs about their respective joints.

1.3 Units

There are two different systems of units which are used for the measurement of kinematic and kinetic variables. They are the English System and the SI (Système International) or Metric System. Each system has two sub-systems and one's choice of sub-system depends upon the size of the variables under consideration. The metric system is more frequently used than the English System and, with a few exceptions, all of the measures referred to in this book are in metric units. For reference purposes, however, all four sets of units for linear and angular variables are presented in Tables 1 and 2 of the Appendix.

2

Linear Motion

2.1 Distance and speed, displacement and velocity

The speed of an object is defined as 'distance travelled per unit of time', or 'the rate of change of distance'.

$$\text{i.e.} \quad \text{Speed} = \frac{\text{distance travelled}}{\text{time}}$$

If distance is measured in miles and time in hours, speed will be in units of miles per hour. For example, if a cross-country runner covers a distance of 10 miles in $\frac{3}{4}$ hour, his or her speed over the 10 miles is given by:

$$\text{Speed} = \frac{\text{Distance}}{\text{time}} = \frac{10\,\text{miles}}{\frac{3}{4}\,\text{hour}} = 13.3\,\text{miles per hour}$$

This is the runner's *average* speed and gives no indication of the variation in his or her running speed over the 10 miles. When the speed of an object is constant over a certain time period, the object is said to move with *uniform* speed. When the speed of an object varies over a certain time period, the object is said to move with *non-uniform* speed.

During a 10 miles cross-country run, the direction of a runner may change many times. In contrast, a 100 metre sprinter runs in a straight line. When the direction as well as the magnitude of the distance travelled and speed of an object is specified, the terms *displacement* and *velocity* are used; displacement indicates distance in a given direction and velocity indicates speed in a given direction. Whereas one might refer to the average speed of a cross-country runner, it would be more appropriate to refer to the average velocity of a 100 metre sprinter.

4

Analysis of the speed of human movement is important in a number of sports; in particular, track athletics and swimming. Knowledge of the average speed and the variation in the speed of an athlete during a race may have important implications for the training of the athlete. For example, an endurance athlete aiming to run 3000 metres in 8 minutes needs to maintain an average speed of 6.25 metres per second (m/s).

$$\text{i.e.} \quad \frac{3000\,\text{metres}}{8 \times 60\,\text{seconds}} = 6.25\,\text{m/s}$$

This means an average lap time of 64 seconds and training would need to be based on this figure.

$$\text{i.e.} \quad \text{average lap time} = \frac{\text{total time}}{\text{no. of laps}}$$

$$= \frac{8 \times 60\,\text{seconds}}{7\tfrac{1}{2}\,\text{laps}}$$

$$= 64\,\text{s per lap}$$

For a sprinter, a knowledge of his or her average speed during a race would be of little value. What may be useful, however, is the variation in the speed of the sprinter during the race. The aim of a sprinter over 100 and 200 m is to achieve maximum speed as soon as possible and maintain it for the remainder of the race. A knowledge of the speed of the sprinter with respect to time during the race could give answers to such questions as,

    (i) How long did it take to achieve maximum speed?

    (ii) How long did the sprinter maintain maximum speed?

    (iii) What was the difference between final and maximum speed?

Such information would undoubtedly have implications for the training of the athlete. In order to obtain a speed–time curve of the sprinter it would first of all be necessary to produce a distance–time curve. The most frequently used method of recording the distance travelled by an object with respect to time is to film the movement of the object. However, in the investigation described below the movement of a sprinter was recorded on videotape. The sprinter, who was a 19-year-old male junior international, was videotaped as he ran 100 metres on a straight level track. Figure 2.1 shows the layout of the camera and other equipment.

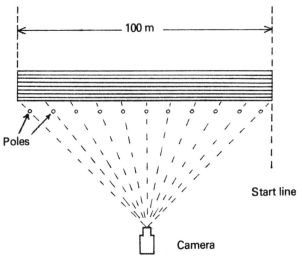

Figure 2.1

Prior to videotaping, the inside of the track, i.e. the lane nearest the camera, was marked off at 10 m intervals from the 100 m start line. The sprinter was then asked to stand at the 10 m mark, i.e. 10 m from the start line. A white pole was then placed approximately 1 m away from the track on a line between the camera lens and the sprinter. This procedure was repeated at each of the other nine 10 m marks, the last one being the finish line. The sprinter was then videotaped as he ran 100 m

Table 2.1

Displacement (m)	Cumulative time (s)	Time for 10 m (s)	Average velocity for 10 m (m/s)
0–10	1.66	1.66	6.03
0–20	2.84	1.18	8.47
0–30	3.88	1.04	9.62
0–40	5.00	1.12	8.92
0–50	5.95	0.95	10.50
0–60	6.97	1.02	9.80
0–70	7.93	0.96	10.40
0–80	8.97	1.04	9.62
0–90	10.07	1.10	9.09
0–100	11.09	1.02	9.80

flat out. By using a stop-watch and playing back the videotape a number of times it was possible to record the time it took the sprinter to run the first 10 m, the first 20 m, the first 30 m etc. up to 100 m. The results are presented in the first two columns of Table 2.1.

This information was then plotted on graph paper to produce the displacement–time curve shown in Figure 2.2. Ideally, the curve should be fairly linear (as in Figure 2.2) and should pass directly through all of the displacement–time points. If a smooth curve cannot be drawn directly through all the displacement–time points, this indicates that the displacement–time data are inaccurate, which is the result of inaccuracy in timing during the recording of the displacement–time data from the video–tape. The only other explanation for a set of displacement–time points which lie on an irregular, wavy curve is that the sprinter was alternatively speeding up and slowing down. This is unlikely to be the case especially during the first 50–60 m when the sprinter is steadily increasing his velocity up to a maximum. Timing distances travelled from videotape is subject to a number of errors which include the quality of the videotape and tape recorder, the quality of the stop-watch and the ability of the investigator to use the stopwatch. In order to obtain a curve which more accurately describes the displacement–time relationship of the sprinter's movement, a 'line of best fit' may be drawn through the set of displacement–time points. The line of best fit is a smooth curve which best represents the 'average' line through the displacement–time points. This technique was used in drawing the curve shown in Figure 2.2; only two points (at 10 and 70 m) lie directly on the curve.

To produce a velocity–time curve of the sprinter's movement, it is necessary to calculate the velocity of the sprinter at different times during the run. This can be done in two ways.

(i) Use of the original displacement–time data. This method would produce 10 velocity–time points representing the average velocity of the sprinter over each successive 10 m of the run. For example,

$$\text{Average velocity over 0–10 m} \quad = \quad \frac{10\,\text{m}}{1.66\,\text{s}} \quad = \quad 6.03\,\text{m/s}$$

$$\text{Average velocity over 10–20 m} \quad = \quad \frac{10\,\text{m}}{1.18\,\text{s}} \quad = \quad 8.47\,\text{m/s}$$

This method has one major disadvantage in that any errors in timing during the recording of the displacement–time data from the video-tape will be greatly exaggerated if the displacement–time data is used to calculate velocity–time data, i.e. the resulting velocity–time curve

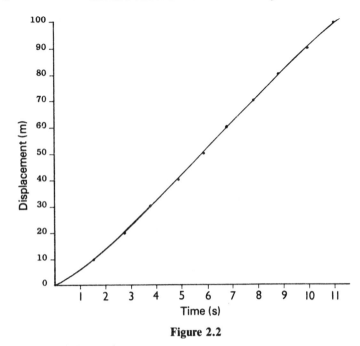

Figure 2.2

will be highly inaccurate. The results of this method are shown in columns 3 and 4 of Table 2.1. If timing had been accurate, the velocity–time data shown in column 4 of Table 2.1 would show a gradual increase over the first 50–60 m followed by a gradual decrease over the latter part of the run. This is not the case, suggesting that at least some of the displacement–time data are inaccurate.

(ii) Use of the displacement–time curve. More accurate velocity–time data will be obtained by using a new set of displacement–time data obtained from the line of best fit displacement–time curve. Instead of finding out the time taken to travel each successive displacement of 10 m, it will ease the calculation of velocity–time data if the displacement–time is recorded in terms of displacement travelled per unit of time. The most convenient interval of time is 1 second. Using the displacement–time curve, parallel lines perpendicular to the time axis are drawn at 1 second intervals such that they intersect the displacement–time curve; see Figure 2.3.

From the points of intersection, another set of parallel lines, perpendicular to the displacement axis, is drawn to intersect the displacement axis. The points of intersection with the displacement axis indicate the

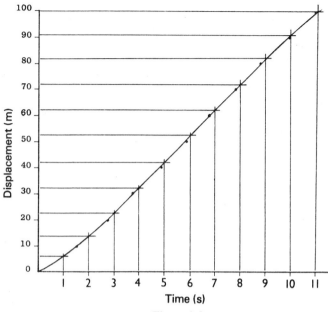

Figure 2.3

cumulative displacement travelled after successive intervals of 1 second; see columns 1 and 2 of Table 2.2. The displacement travelled in each 1 second interval and, therefore, the average velocity of the sprinter during each 1 second interval after the start of the run can then

Table 2.2

Time interval (s)	Cumulative displacement (m)	Displacement travelled in time interval (m)	Average velocity in time interval (m/s)
0–1	5.00	5.00	5.00
1–2	12.75	7.75	7.75
2–3	21.75	9.00	9.00
3–4	31.00	9.25	9.25
4–5	40.75	9.75	9.75
5–6	50.75	10.00	10.00
6–7	60.75	10.00	10.00
7–8	70.75	10.00	10.00
8–9	80.50	9.75	9.75
9–10	90.00	9.50	9.50
10–11	99.40	9.40	9.40

be obtained; see columns 3 and 4 of Table 2.2. Unlike the velocity–time data obtained directly from the original displacement–time data (column 4, Table 2.1), the velocity–time data obtained from the line of best fit displacement–time curve (column 4, Table 2.2) shows that the velocity of the sprinter increased fairly smoothly to a maximum value and then gradually decreased; this is typical of the smooth nature of maximum effort sprinting, especially over 100 m.

The velocity–time data obtained from the displacement–time curve is presented in Figure 2.4 together with the 'line of best fit' velocity–time curve of the sprinter's movement. Since the velocity–time data represent average velocities, each point is plotted at the mid-point of the interval to which it refers. The displacement–time curve is also shown in Figure 2.4 in order to aid the analysis of the motion. It can be seen that the velocity of the sprinter increased very rapidly during the first second of motion (5.0 m). During the next 4¼ seconds the velocity gradually increased to a maximum value of about 10 m/s which was achieved at about 50 m. Maximum velocity was maintained for about 1 second (50–60 m) and then decreased steadily from 10 m/s to around 9.2 m/s during the last 40 m.

In order to show that the displacement–time and velocity–time

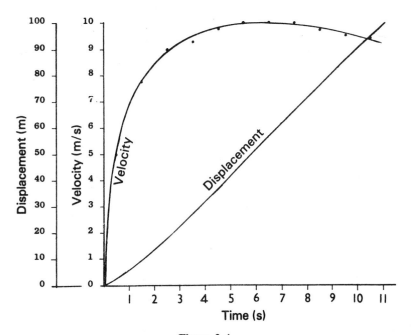

Figure 2.4

curves shown in Figure 2.4 were truly representative of the sprinter's pattern of motion over 100 m it would be necessary to produce displacement–time and velocity–time curves from a number of runs, not just one as described here. However, if Figure 2.4 is assumed to be the end result of such a procedure, the curves would suggest that in training particular emphasis should be placed on improving the sprinter's ability to maintain maximum velocity for a longer period of time. Figure 2.4 shows that the sprinter covered the last 40 m in about 4.35 s (average velocity = 9.19 m/s). If the sprinter could have maintained the maximum velocity of 10 m/s till the end of the run, he could have covered the last 40 m in 4.0 s, i.e. a saving of 0.35 s. This could make the difference between success and failure in a race. In order to make other inferences regarding the velocity–time characteristics of the sprinter at different stages in the 100 m run – such as the start, pick-up, period of maximum velocity and finish – it would be necessary to compare his or her velocity–time curve with that of a top-class sprinter.

2.2 Acceleration

The acceleration of an object is defined as 'change in velocity per unit of time' or 'the rate of change of velocity'.

$$\text{i.e.} \quad \text{acceleration} \quad = \quad \frac{v - u}{t_2 - t_1}$$

where

$$u \quad = \quad \text{velocity of object at time } t_1$$

and

$$v \quad = \quad \text{velocity of object at some later time } t_2$$

When the velocity of an object increases during a particular period of time, the acceleration of the object is said to be positive. When the velocity of an object decreases during a particular period of time the acceleration of the object is said to be negative. Negative acceleration is often referred to as deceleration.

The velocity–time curve of the sprinter shown in Figure 2.4 shows that the velocity of the sprinter 7 s after the start of the run was 10.00 m/s. Since his velocity at the start of the run was zero, his average acceleration during the first 7 s of motion is given by,

$$\text{Acceleration} \quad = \quad \frac{10.00 - 0}{7 - 0} \quad = \quad 1.43 \text{ metres per second per second}$$

i.e. his velocity increased at an average of 1.43 m/s for every second of motion. The velocity of the sprinter 11 s after the start was 9.21 m/s. Therefore, his average acceleration during the period 7 to 11 s after the start is given by,

$$\text{Acceleration} = \frac{9.21 - 10.00}{11 - 7} = -0.19 \text{ metres per second per second}$$

The negative sign indicates that the sprinter was decelerating during the period of time under consideration, i.e. his velocity decreased by an average of 0.19 m/s for each second between 7 and 11 s after the start of the run. The units 'metres per second per second' are usually written m/s^2. Column 2 of Table 2.3 presents the velocity of the sprinter after each second. The velocity data are taken from the velocity–time curve shown in Figure 2.4. Column 3 of Table 2.3 presents the change in velocity during each second of motion, which in this case is the same as the acceleration of the sprinter as shown in column 4 of Table 2.3. The acceleration–time data are plotted in Figure 2.5 together with 'line of best fit' acceleration–time curve, the velocity–time curve, and the displacement–time curve.

The acceleration–time curve shows that the sprinter's acceleration was positive for approximately $6\frac{1}{2}$ s after the start of the run, i.e. his velocity continued to increase during this period up to a maximum of about 10.00 m/s. During the remainder of the run, acceleration was negative, i.e., velocity gradually decreased.

Table 2.3

Time interval (s)	Cumulative velocity (m/s)	Change in velocity per second (m/s)	Acceleration (m/s^2)
0–1	6.65	6.65	6.65
1–2	8.37	1.72	1.72
2–3	9.17	0.80	0.80
3–4	9.62	0.45	0.45
4–5	9.88	0.26	0.26
5–6	10.00	0.12	0.12
6–7	10.00	0.00	0.00
7–8	9.90	−0.10	−0.10
8–9	9.70	−0.20	−0.20
9–10	9.46	−0.24	−0.24
10–11	9.21	−0.25	−0.25

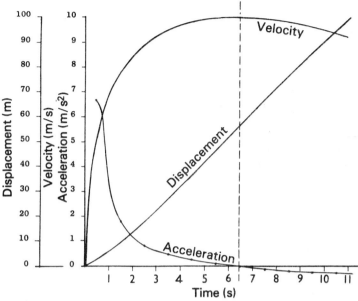

Figure 2.5

2.3 Vector and scalar quantities

All of the variables mentioned in this book can be classified into two groups. Variables such as distance and speed which can be completely specified in terms of *magnitude* (size) are called scalar quantities. Variables such as displacement and velocity which require specification in both *magnitude and direction* are called vector quantities. A vector is simply a straight line which represents a particular variable in magnitude (length of line) and direction. Other examples of scalar and vector quantities are listed below.

Scalar quantities	*Vector quantities*
Volume	Acceleration
Area	Force
Time	
Temperature	
Mass	

The application of vectors in movement analysis will now be described with reference to displacement, velocity and force.

2.3.1 Displacement vectors

If we are told that a man runs 3 miles then walks 2 miles, we know that
he has travelled a distance of 5 miles but we have no idea where the man
is in relation to his starting point since we do not know the directions
in which he ran and walked. If we are given the directions as well as
how far he travelled, we are then dealing with vector quantities, i.e.
displacements, and can find out where the man is at the end of his
journey. For example, suppose that starting from a point A, the man
runs 3 miles due north to a point B, then walks 2 miles due east to a point
C; the two displacements can be represented by vectors $\overline{AB}$ and $\overline{BC}$ as
shown in Figure 2.6. The point C can be specified by measuring the
distance AC and the angle θ;

$$AC \;=\; 3.6\,cm \;\equiv\; 3.6\,miles$$
$$\theta \;=\; 33°$$

i.e. in relation to the point A, the point C can be specified by the vector
sum of $\overline{AB} + \overline{BC}$ or by the single vector $\overline{AC}$ (3.6 miles N 33° E). Vector
addition is clearly not the same as arithmetic (or scalar) addition. The
resultant of the displacements 3 miles north and 2 miles due east is
3.6 miles N 33° E. The resultant of the distances 3 miles and 2 miles is
5 miles. Since $\overline{AC}$ is the result of $\overline{AB} + \overline{BC}$ it is called a *resultant vector*
and $\overline{AB}$ and $\overline{BC}$ are called *component vectors*. $\overline{AC}$ is, in fact, the
resultant displacement of the man from the point A.

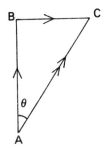

scale: 1 cm ≡ 1 mile
$\overline{AB}$ = 3 miles due north
$\overline{BC}$ = 2 miles due east
$\overline{AC}$ = 3.6 miles N 33° E

Figure 2.6

Irrespective of the number of component vectors used to describe the
motion of a particular object, the net result of all the component vectors can be specified by a *single resultant vector*. For example suppose
the man in the above example walked a further 2 miles due south from

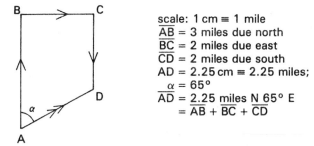

Figure 2.7

the point C to a point D. We now have a third component vector $\overline{CD}$. The point D can be specified by the resultant vector $\overline{AD}$ as shown in Figure 2.7.

2.3.2 Velocity vectors
If a ship without a keel starts to sail due north in a wind blowing due west, the resultant velocity (speed and direction) of the ship will be specified by the resultant of:

(a) the velocity V_1 of the ship caused by the drive of its engines (speed) and rudder (direction)
and

(b) the velocity V_2 of the ship imparted to it by the wind.

If $V_1 = 10$ knots due north and $V_2 = 5$ knots due west, the resultant velocity of the ship can be found as shown in Figure 2.8. A vector $\overline{AB}$ is drawn to represent V_1. Starting at B, a vector BC is drawn to represent V_2. The resultant of V_1 and V_2 is the vector $\overline{AC}$, i.e. the vector

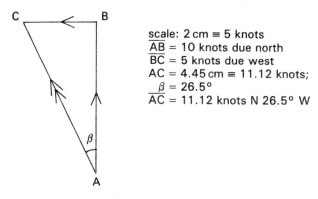

Figure 2.8

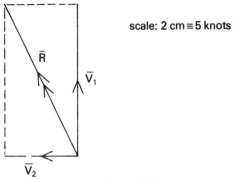

scale: 2 cm ≡ 5 knots

Figure 2.9

running from the starting point of vector $\overline{AB}$ to the end point of vector $\overline{BC}$. This method of obtaining the resultant of two or more vectors is called the vector chain method. There is another method called the parallelogram of vectors which is useful when there are only two component vectors but rather laborious when there are three or more component vectors. In this method any two component vectors form two adjacent sides of a parallelogram. The resultant of the two component vectors is given by the length and direction of the diagonal of the parallelogram between the two component vectors. In the above example of the ship, $V_1 = 10$ knots due north and $V_2 = 5$ knots due west. The resultant of V_1 and V_2 is found by the parallelogram of vectors method as shown in Figure 2.9. In this case the parallelogram is a rectangle since the component vectors are at right angles to each other. If the wind was blowing S 60° W such that V_2 was 5 knots S 60° W the resultant velocity of the ship would be 8.8 knots N 30° W as shown in Figure 2.10.

When using the parallelogram of vectors method to find the resultant

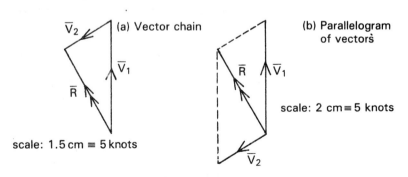

Figure 2.10

(a) No cross-wind   **(b) Cross-wind**   **(c) Cross-wind**

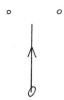

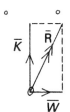

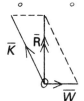

Figure 2.11

of three or more component vectors, a first step is to find the resultant R_1 of any two component vectors. R_1 is then 'added' to a third component vector and the process is repeated with a fourth and subsequent component vectors until one vector remains, i.e. the resultant of all the component vectors.

Imagine the situation of a rugby player attempting to convert the ball from a place kick. Provided that there is no cross-wind blowing the kicker has only to kick the ball in the direction of the middle of the posts; see Figure 2.11(a). If there is a cross-wind, however, the motion of the ball will be the result of,

(i) the velocity K of the ball imparted to it by the kick,

and

(ii) the velocity W of the ball imparted to it by the wind.

If the kicker does not take account of the wind, the ball will not travel in the direction of the middle of the posts; see Figure 2.11(b). A good kicker will take account of the wind such that the combined effects of his kick and the wind direct the ball between the posts; see Figure 2.11(c). The ball does not travel in a straight line but along a curve, as shown in Figure 2.12. Assuming that the wind continues to blow throughout the period of ball flight, the speed of the ball imparted by the wind will gradually increase during the flight. However, the speed of the ball imparted by the kick will decrease gradually during the flight due to air resistance. Consequently, the direction of the ball will continuously change as shown in Figure 2.12. In this example it is assumed that the kick does not impart spin to the ball. The mechanics of the flight of a spinning ball are more complex than for a non-spinning ball.

2.3.3 Force vectors

Force is a vector quantity since it has magnitude and direction. Consider two men pushing a box across a gymnasium floor as in Figure 2.13(a). The effect of the two forces A and B will be the same as that

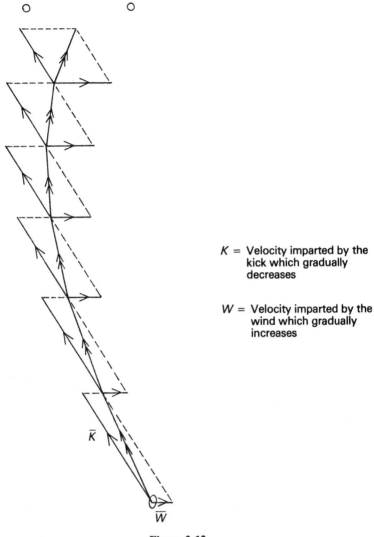

K = Velocity imparted by the kick which gradually decreases

W = Velocity imparted by the wind which gradually increases

Figure 2.12

of a single force R, i.e. the resultant of the two forces, such that the box will move in the direction of R; see Figure 2.13(b). In a tug-of-war contest the force exerted on the rope by either team is equal to the resultant of all the individual forces exerted by the members of the team; see Figure 2.14. The team which can pull the hardest, i.e. exert the most force on the rope, will win the contest. For example, consider

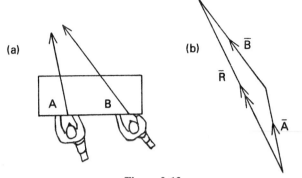

Figure 2.13

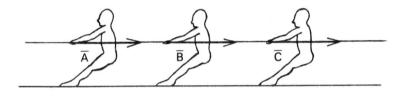

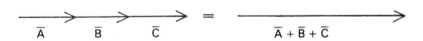

Figure 2.14

two teams of three pulling against each other as in Figure 2.15 where the forces exerted by the individual contestants are represented by individual vectors. If the total force exerted on the rope by team 1 $(A + B + C)$ is greater than that exerted by team 2 $(D + E + F)$ there will be a resultant force acting on the rope in the direction of team 1; see Figure 2.16.

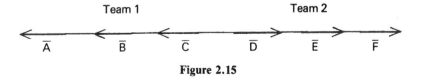

Figure 2.15

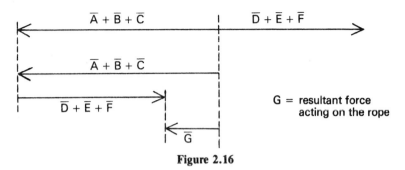

Figure 2.16

In comparison with the forces exerted on the rope by the two teams, the resultant force acting on the rope may be very small such that the speed of movement of the rope towards either team's area will be very small. When both teams exert the same amount of force, the resultant force on the rope will be zero and the rope will not move at all.

When more than two non-parallel forces act on an object, the resultant of all the forces can be found by applying the one-stage vector chain method or the parallelogram of vectors method in two or more stages. For example, consider the situation of three men pushing a car which is represented in Figure 2.17(a). The vector chain solution is shown in Figure 2.17(b).

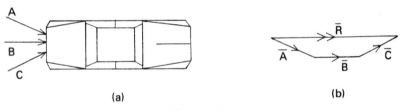

Figure 2.17

The parallelogram of vectors method is a two-stage process. Stage one involves finding the resultant R_1 of two of the forces. The second stage involves finding the resultant of R_1 and the third force; see Figure 2.18.

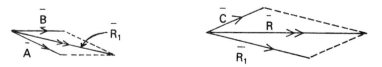

Figure 2.18

2.4   Mass, inertia and linear momentum

The mass of an object is the quantity of matter of which an object is composed and depends upon the density and volume of the object. If the density of two objects is the same, the one with the larger volume will have the greater mass. The mass of an object is constant wherever it happens to be in the universe. In the metric system mass is measured in either grams (g) or kilograms (kg). An object at rest has a certain reluctance to do anything other than remain at rest. This reluctance to start moving is referred to as the *inertia* of the object. The mass of an object is a direct measure of the inertia of the object. The greater the mass of an object, the greater will be its reluctance to start moving, i.e. the greater will be its inertia. For example, the inertia of a stationary soccer ball (a small mass) is small in comparison with the inertia of a heavy barbell (a large mass), i.e. far less effort is required to move the ball than the barbell.

Just as an object at rest exhibits a reluctance to start moving, a moving object exhibits a reluctance to do anything other than continue to move in the direction in which it is already moving. For example, anyone who has ever been hit by a hockey or cricket ball will recall that the ball exhibited a great resistance to alter its speed and direction of movement!

In comparison with the inertia of a resting object, however, the reluctance of an object to alter its speed and direction of movement depends not only on the mass of the object but also on its velocity. The product of the mass of an object and its velocity is called the linear momentum or 'quantity of motion' of the object. For example, the linear momentum of a rugby player of mass 70 kg moving with a velocity of 5 m/s is given by,

$$70\,\text{kg} \times 5\,\text{m/s} \quad = \quad 350\,\text{kg m/s}$$

In sports situations the mass of a player is constant, if the loss of mass due to the exercise is discounted, and his or her momentum will vary directly with velocity. In rugby football, for example, a well-used ploy is to set up a situation in which the ball can be passed to a player who is moving forward very quickly close to the opposition goal line, since the faster the player is moving on receiving the ball the greater will be the player's momentum and the more difficult it will be for the opposition to stop that player.

2.5   Force and Newton's First Law of Motion

An object at rest will begin to move only when it is acted upon by an unbalanced force, i.e. when it experiences a push or pull. Furthermore, an object moving with uniform velocity (i.e. in a straight line with constant speed) will

(a) change direction,
or (b) be speeded up, i.e. accelerated,
or (c) be slowed down, i.e. decelerated,

only when it is acted upon by an unbalanced force. Force is that which alters or tends to alter an object's state of rest or uniform velocity. This phenomenon was observed by Sir Isaac Newton (1642–1727) and formed the basis of the first of his three Laws of Motion. The law, which is sometimes referred to as the law of inertia, may be expressed as follows:

Every object will remain at rest or continue with uniform velocity unless acted upon by an unbalanced force.

Two examples will serve to illustrate the operation of the law.

(i) At the start of a soccer match, a player must kick (apply force to) the ball in order to get it moving.
(ii) A person travelling on a bus will be moving with the same velocity as the bus. If the velocity of the bus is suddenly reduced by braking or a collision, there will be a tendency for that person, who is not 'attached' to the bus, to be thrown forward since he or she will still tend to move forward with the velocity possessed before the bus braked. Seat belts are worn by passengers in motor cars and other vehicles in order to prevent injury which might otherwise result from sharp changes in the velocity of the vehicle.

There are two kinds of forces, contact forces and attraction forces. There is only one attraction force which affects human movement, i.e. the force of attraction exerted by the earth on every object at or close to the earth's surface. This force is considered in detail in Section 2.6 which concerns Newton's Law of Gravitation. All other forces which affect human movement are contact forces. Contact forces result from physical contact between different objects. The force generated between two objects which come into contact with each other is normally in the form of a push (compression) or a pull (tension). For example:

(a) Pushing or pulling open a door which would otherwise remain closed.
(b) Trapping or laying-off a soccer ball.
(c) Hitting a tennis ball.
(d) Pulling on a rope in order to bring down a beam in the gymnasium.

Not all forces produce or alter motion. Whether a particular force has any effect on the motion of an object depends on the size of the force in relation to the object. For example, in order to lift a particular object, such as a barbell, the lifter must exert a force greater than the weight of the barbell. He or she can apply force to the bar but unless the force applied is greater than the weight of the bar the latter will not leave the floor.

A force which acts on, or is applied to an object by an agency outside the object itself is called an *external* force. The action of kicking a football, throwing a javelin, or pushing in a rugby scrum are examples of external forces acting on, or being applied to objects, i.e. to a ball, javelin and scrum respectively. An *internal* force is a force which results from actions within the object itself. The actions of muscles pulling on their attachments within the human body are examples of internal forces.

We shall see later that the relatively simple act of walking from one place to another across a room is made possible only by the interaction of internal forces resulting from muscular contractions *within the body* and the external forces of body weight and friction, acting *on the body*.

2.6 Newton's Law of Gravitation (Law of Attraction); Gravity and Weight

There is a well-known story about Sir Isaac Newton who, it is said, was sitting under an apple tree one day when he saw an apple fall from a tree. This observation formed the basis of what has come to be known as Newton's Law of Gravitation (or Law of Attraction) which states that:

> *Every object (particle of matter, body) attracts every other object with a force which varies directly with the product of the masses of the objects and inversely with the square of the distance between them.*

Thus the force of attraction, F, which exists between two objects of masses m_1 and m_2 at a distance $d*$ apart is given by,

$$F = \frac{Gm_1m_2}{d^2} \tag{1}$$

where G is a constant known as the Constant of Gravitation. In very simple terms the Law of Gravitation means that the force of attraction between any pair of objects will be greater the larger the masses of the objects and the closer the objects are together.

---

* d is specifically the distance between the individual centres of mass of the two objects.

It is, perhaps, a little hard to appreciate that a force of attraction exists between *any* pair of objects. However, the force of attraction between any two objects on or close to the surface of the earth is so minute that it does not cause the objects to move towards each other. For example, the force of attraction between two men each of mass 70 kg and standing 50 cm apart is approximately one ten-millionth of a kilogram weight ($1/10^7$ kg wt). This force of attraction becomes even smaller the further apart the men move.

There is, however, one object which does exert a significant force of attraction on every other object. This special object is the earth. In relation to the Law of Gravitation the earth is simply a very large object. The earth has a huge mass and even though the distance between the centre of the earth and any object on the surface of the earth (or in space close to the surface of the earth) is extremely large, the force of attraction between the earth and any object is much larger than that which exists between any two objects on or close to the earth's surface. This force of attraction between the earth and any other object is not large enough to have any effect on the movement of the earth but is certainly large enough to pull any other object towards the earth. For example, consider two light bulbs hanging from separate flexes a few feet apart on the same ceiling. By the Law of Gravitation there will be a force of attraction exerted between each light bulb and the earth, such that each light bulb and flex hang vertically. There will also be a force of attraction exerted between the two light bulbs. However, the magnitude of this force of attraction is insignificant and the light bulbs continue to hang vertically rather than angled towards each other.

The force of attraction which the earth exerts on any object is known as the *weight* of the object. This is the force which keeps a man in contact with the earth or brings him back to the surface of the earth very quickly should he momentarily leave it as, for example, when jumping off the ground. By using the Law of Gravitation, the weight W of an object O may be expressed thus:

$$W = \frac{Gm_o m_e}{d^2} \tag{2}$$

where

$$
\begin{aligned}
W &= \text{Weight of object} \\
G &= \text{Gravitational constant} \\
m_o &= \text{Mass of the object} \\
m_e &= \text{Mass of the earth} \\
d &= \text{Radius of the earth*}
\end{aligned}
$$

* The distance between the surface of the earth and the centre of mass of the object is infinitesimal in comparison with d and is, therefore, not included in the expression.

Since G and m_e are constants, the term Gm_e/d^2 is constant for any point on the earth's surface, i.e.

$$W = m_o g \tag{3}$$

where

$$g = \frac{Gm_e}{d^2} \tag{4}$$

'g', not to be confused with G, is referred to as *gravity*. The earth is not a perfect sphere, d being slightly greater at the equator than at the poles. Since g varies inversely with the square of d, g is slightly greater at the poles than at the equator. It follows that the weight of an object, i.e. the force an object exerts due to gravity, will be slightly greater at the poles than at the equator. The Law of Gravitation applies not only to the earth but also to all the other planets of the solar system. Since the masses and radii of the individual planets differ from each other it follows that the weight of an object on one planet will be different from its weight on every other planet. For example, the mass of the moon is approximately 1/81 of that of the earth and the radius of the moon is approximately 7/25 of that of the earth. The weight of an object on the moon can be expressed as follows:

$$W_n = \frac{Gm_o m_n}{d_n^2} \tag{5}$$

where

$$
\begin{aligned}
W_n &= \text{Weight of the object on the moon} \\
m_o &= \text{Mass of the object} \\
m_n &= \text{Mass of the moon} \\
d_n &= \text{Radius of the moon}
\end{aligned}
$$

but

$$m_n = \frac{m_e}{81} \qquad \text{where } m_e = \text{mass of the earth}$$

and

$$d_n = \frac{7d_e}{25} \qquad \text{where } d_e = \text{radius of the earth}$$

By substituting for m_n and d_n in equation (5) we obtain:

$$W_n \;=\; \frac{Gm_o \left(\dfrac{m_e}{81}\right)}{\left(\dfrac{7d_e}{25}\right)^2} \;\simeq\; \frac{1}{6}\left(\frac{Gm_o m_e}{d_e^2}\right) \tag{6}$$

but

$$W_o \;=\; \frac{Gm_o m_e}{d_e^2} \tag{7}$$

where W_o = weight of the same object on earth. Therefore, from equations (6) and (7),

$$W_n \;\simeq\; \frac{W_o}{6}$$

i.e., the weight of the object on the moon is approximately one sixth of its weight on earth. Since the mass of the object is constant, it follows that the moon's gravity is approximately one sixth of the earth's gravity. This can be clearly demonstrated by manipulating equation (6) as follows:

$$\text{From equation (6)} \qquad W_n \;=\; m_o \left(\frac{Gm_e}{6d_e^2}\right) \;=\; m_o g_n$$

where

$$g_n \;=\; \text{the moon's gravity} \;=\; \frac{Gm_e}{6d_e^2} \tag{8}$$

From equations (4) and (8),

$$g_n \;=\; \frac{g}{6}$$

where g is the earth's gravity. The reader will no doubt remember the ease of movement experienced by those astronauts who landed on the moon. The reasons for this ease of movement are two-fold.

(i) The strength of a particular astronaut would be the same as it would be on earth, but his weight would be approximately one sixth of his earth weight. Therefore, he could project himself off the surface of the moon far more easily than he could project himself off the surface of the earth.

(ii) The astronaut would be attracted back to the surface of the moon by a force of approximately one sixth of the attraction force on earth; consequently, he would appear to float down to the surface of the moon rather than fall rapidly as he would on earth.

2.7 Newton's second law of motion; the impulse of a force

From Newton's first law of motion it follows that in order to change the velocity of an object, i.e. to accelerate or decelerate an object, an unbalanced force must be applied to the object. Any change in the velocity of an object will result simultaneously in a change in the momentum of the object. When a force acts on an object the change in momentum, i.e. increase or decrease, experienced by the object depends upon the size of the force and the duration for which the force acts. It was this observation which led Newton to formulate the second of his laws of motion. This law, sometimes referred to as the law of momentum, may be expressed as follows.

When a force acts on an object the change in momentum experienced by the object takes place in the direction of the force and is proportional to the size of the force and the duration for which the force acts.

$$\text{i.e.} \quad Ft \propto mv - mu \qquad (1)$$

where

F = magnitude of applied force
t = duration of force application
m = mass of the object
u = velocity of object immediately prior to force application
v = velocity of object immediately after removal of the force

$$\text{From (1)} \quad F \propto \frac{mv - mu}{t} \qquad (2)$$

The law is often expressed in terms of equation (2) as follows:

When a force acts on an object the rate of change of momentum experienced by the object is proportional to the size of the force and takes place in the direction of the force.

To illustrate the operation of this law consider a soccer ball on the penalty spot. Before the kick is taken the momentum of the ball is zero since it has mass but no velocity. As the kick is taken, force is applied to the ball for as long as the ball is in contact with the kicker's boot. When the ball breaks contact with the kicker's boot it has velocity, and, therefore, a certain momentum. Using equation (2) above,

$$F \propto \frac{mv - mu}{t}$$

where

$$
\begin{aligned}
F &= \text{average force applied to the ball during the kick} \\
t &= \text{duration of time that the ball was in contact with} \\
  & \quad \text{the ball, i.e. the amount of time that force was} \\
  & \quad \text{being applied to the ball} \\
m &= \text{mass of the ball} \\
u \text{ and } v &= \text{velocity of ball immediately before and after the} \\
  & \quad \text{kick, respectively.}
\end{aligned}
$$

In this particular example, $u = 0$, such that:

$$F \propto \frac{mv}{t}$$

Since $v/t = a$ = average acceleration of the ball while in contact with the kicker's boot, it follows that,

$$F \propto ma \qquad (3)$$

In examples where u is not zero,

$$F \propto \frac{m(v-u)}{t}$$

i.e.　　$F \propto ma$　　　　where　　$a = \frac{v-u}{t}$

From equation (3)

$$a \propto \frac{F}{m} \qquad (4)$$

Newton's second law is sometimes expressed in terms of equation (4) as follows:

> *The acceleration experienced by an object when acted upon by a force is directly proportional to the size of the force, inversely proportional to the mass of the object and takes place in the direction of the force.*

Consequently, the greater the force applied to an object, the greater will be the acceleration of the object, and the greater will be the velocity of the object when the force is removed. For example, the harder a soccer player kicks a ball (i.e. the more force he applies) the greater will be the velocity of the ball when it leaves his foot. Similarly, the more force that a shot putter can apply to the shot before release the greater will be the velocity of the shot at release and, other things being equal such as the height of release and angle of trajectory, the further the shot will travel. However, from Newton's second law (see equation (1)) the amount by which the velocity of an object can be increased depends not only on the size of the force applied but also on the length of time that the force can be applied. It follows, therefore, that in order to give an object, such as a shot, maximum velocity it is necessary to apply as much force as possible for as long as possible. When a force is applied to an object the product of the force and the length of time that the force is applied is called the impulse of the force, i.e.

$$\text{force} \times \text{time} \quad = \quad \text{impulse of force}$$

The application of the impulse principle has led to the development of sports techniques, particularly in throwing events. Consider the shot putt, for example. The amount of force that the athlete can apply to the shot depends very much on his strength. Generally speaking the stronger the athlete the greater the amount of force he will be able to apply.

The length of time that the athlete can apply force to the shot, however, depends entirely on the shot-putt technique employed. Originally the technique consisted of a standing putt; see Figure 2.19(e–g). The development of the technique has resulted from attempts to utilise the rear part of the shot putt circle in order to apply force to the shot for a longer period of time (and over a greater distance) prior to release. In 1952 at the Helsinki Olympic Games the winner of the shot putt, Parry O'Brien of USA, demonstrated a new technique which has since been used by every other Olympic champion and world-record holder. The technique involves basically three stages. The athlete takes up a position in the rear part of the circle with the big toe of the right foot (for a right-handed thrower) up against the inner side

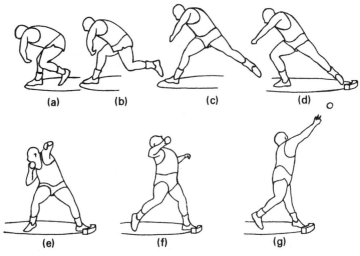

Figure 2.19

of the circle. From this position the athlete flexes his or her hips and knees such that the shot may actually be outside the back of the circle; see Figure 2.19(a). From this position the movement across the circle is initiated by an explosive extension of the left leg, closely followed by, and in association with, extension of the right knee; see Figure 2.19(b) and (c). The purpose of this movement is to generate velocity in the shot in the direction of the putt. Prior to landing with the left foot close to the stopboard, the athlete flexes the right knee and moves the right foot underneath his or her body such that it lands about half way across the circle; see Figure 2.19(d). At this stage the athlete is close to a position from which the final putting movement, basically a standing throw, can be made. The advantage of the O'Brien technique is that as a result of the impulse of the force applied to the shot in the movement across the circle, the shot will be moving fairly quickly in the direction of the putt before the final putting movement is initiated. Consequently the total impulse applied to the shot during the complete sequence of movements will be considerably greater than that applied in a standing putt, and the greater will be the velocity of the shot at release. The technique of discus throwing originally consisted of a standing throw, i.e. half a turn which was made from the front of the circle; see Figure 2.20(f–i). Nowadays the most popular technique involves one and three-quarter turns with the athlete starting from a position in the back of the circle and facing in the opposite direction to that of the throw. The athlete starts the turning movement from a position with the shoulders turned as far as possible to the right (for a right-handed thrower); see

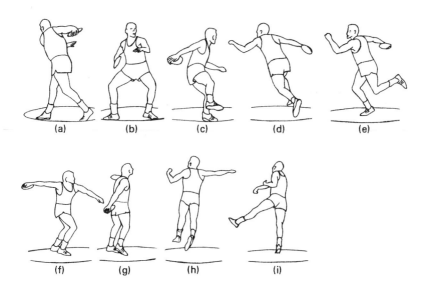

Figure 2.20

Figure 2.20(a). The athlete then turns to his or her left and performs a running-like movement across the circle which brings him or her into a position from which the final slinging action can be initiated. The impulse of the force applied to the discus using the one and three-quarter turns technique is much greater than that in a half-turn standing throw and consequently the greater will be the release velocity of the discus. In recent years some shot putters have been experimenting with the one and three-quarter turns discus technique and there is evidence to suggest that it may be superior to the O'Brien technique of shot putting; see Figure 2.21.

2.8 Units of force

From Newton's Second Law of Motion, the relationship between the acceleration a experienced by a mass m when acted upon by a force F is given by,

$$F \propto ma$$

Therefore,

$$F = Kma \qquad (1)$$

where K is a constant of proportionality.

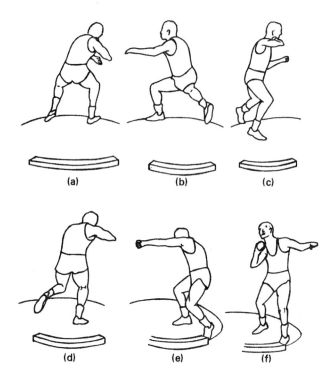

Figure 2.21

In the metric system, one of the two units of force is the newton. A newton (N) is defined as the force acting on a mass of 1 kg which gives it an acceleration of $1 \, \text{m/s}^2$. By substituting $F = 1 \, \text{N}$, $m = 1 \, \text{kg}$ and $a = 1 \, \text{m/s}^2$ in (1), we obtain $K = 1$.

$$\text{i.e.} \quad F = ma \quad (2)$$

The dyne is the other unit of force in the metric system. It is defined as the force acting on a mass of 1 g which gives it an acceleration of $1 \, \text{cm/s}^2$. It was shown in Section 2.6 that the weight W of an object of mass m is given by

$$W = mg \quad (3)$$

where g is gravity. It follows from equations (2) and (3) that gravity is an acceleration. The magnitude of gravity varies slightly at different points on the earth's surface (see Section 2.6), with an average value of 9.81 m/s². Therefore, an object falling freely under gravity undergoes an acceleration of 9.81 m/s² as long as it is not moving rapidly enough for air resistance to become appreciable (see example of skydiver, p. 36).

From equation (2) the weight of a mass of 1 kg (1 kg wt) is given by

$$1 \text{ kg wt} = 1 \text{ kg} \times 9.81 \text{ m/s}^2$$
$$= 9.81 \text{ kg m/s}^2 = 9.81 \text{ N}$$

The kg wt is a gravitational unit of force and most weighing machines in everyday use, for example, kitchen scales, bathroom scales and shop scales, are graduated in kg wt. Thus if a man of mass 70 kg stood on a set of bathroom scales, he would see that his weight was 70 kg wt. This weight is equivalent to 686 N.

$$\text{i.e. from} \quad F = ma,$$
$$70 \text{ kg wt} = 70 \text{ kg} \times 9.81 \text{ m/s}^2$$
$$= 686 \text{ N}$$

In mathematical calculations using metric units, force will be in newtons. For example, consider the force acting on a soccer ball of mass 0.3 kg during a goal kick. The velocity u of the ball before the kick would be zero. If the velocity v of the ball immediately after the kick was 40 m/s and the time of contact t between the kicker's boot and the ball was 0.05 s, the average force F exerted on the ball could be calculated by applying Newton's Second Law of Motion as follows:

$$F = \frac{m(v-u)}{t}$$
$$= \frac{0.3(40-0)}{0.05}$$
$$= 240 \text{ N}$$

Since 1 kg wt = 9.81 N,

$$F = \frac{240}{9.81} \text{ kg wt} = 24.4 \text{ kg wt}$$

As a further illustration, consider the force acting on a golf ball during a drive.

If mass of ball = 0.06 kg

$$u = 0$$
$$v = 70 \text{ m/s}$$
$$t = 0.0005 \text{ s} \quad \text{(between clubhead and ball)},$$

the average force F acting on the ball during impact is given by,

$$F = \frac{m(v-u)}{t}$$

$$= \frac{0.06(70-0)}{0.0005}$$

$$= 8400 \text{ N}$$

$$= \frac{8400}{9.81} \text{kg wt} = 856 \text{ kg wt}$$

In addition to the kg wt, there is another much older gravitational unit of weight, i.e., the lb wt (pound weight; see Appendix, Table 1). Since 1 kg wt = 2.2 lb wt, the force on the golf ball in the above example may be given as 1882 lb wt; i.e.

$$F = 856 \times 2.2 = 1882 \text{ lb wt}$$

Furthermore, since 2240 lb wt = 1 tn wt (ton weight)

$$F = \frac{1882}{2240} \text{tn wt} = 0.85 \text{ tn wt}$$

2.9 The free body diagram

A sketch showing, in vector form, all of the forces acting on an object is called a *free body diagram*. The forces represented may be contact forces such as pulls, pushes, support forces, wind resistance and buoyancy effects, or attraction forces such as gravitational force (weight) and magnetism. For example, the only forces acting on a man standing upright will be the weight of his body W, and the support force R which is exerted by the floor on the man in order to counteract W; see Figure 2.22(a). In a free body diagram the point of application of a force may be indicated by either the tail end or the arrow of the vector

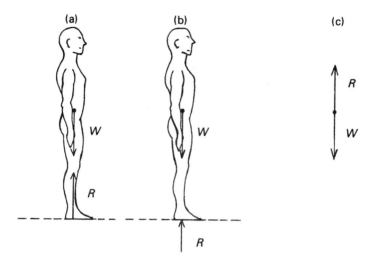

Figure 2.22

representing the force; see R in Figures 2.22(a) and (b). When only the linear effect of the forces acting on an object is required, rather than both the linear and angular effects, the free body diagram may be simplified by representing the object as a spot from which the various force vectors arise; see Figure 2.22(c).

2.10 Resultant force and equilibrium

An object at rest is acted on by at least two forces. One force acting on the object will be the weight of the object. Since the object is at rest the weight of the object must be balanced by a force equal in magnitude but opposite in direction, such that the combined effect of both forces, i.e. the resultant or net force acting on the object, is zero. For example, when a man is standing upright as in Figure 2.22 the support force, R, is equal in magnitude but opposite in direction to the weight of the man. If the man stood on a tightrope as in Figure 2.23 the weight of his body would be supported by the combined effect of the forces exerted in each part of the rope.

Irrespective of the number of forces acting on an object, if the object is at rest the resultant of all the forces must be zero. The resultant force acting on an object moving with uniform velocity (i.e., constant speed in a straight line) is also zero. It is only when the resultant of all the forces acting on an object is greater than zero that the object will begin to move or change its motion from a state of uniform velocity. When the resultant force acting on an object is zero, the object is said to be in a state of *equilibrium*. Therefore, Newton's First Law of Motion could be rephrased as follows:

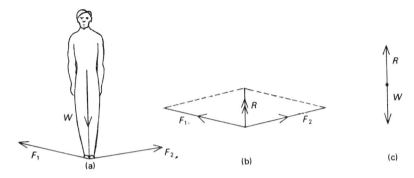

Figure 2.23

> *Every object will remain in equilibrium unless the result-
> ant force acting on the object is greater than zero.*

To illustrate further the concepts of resultant force and equilibrium
consider the motion of (a) a skydiver; and (b) a man travelling in a lift.

2.10.1 Skydiver

When the skydiver jumps out of an aeroplane he or she is accelerated
towards the earth by the force of body weight; see Figure 2.24(a). For
the first few seconds of the fall he or she will experience a uniform
downward acceleration, i.e. gravity. However, as downward velocity
increases so does the upthrust of air on the underside of the body, i.e.
the air resistance. After about 5 seconds, when downward velocity is
approximately 50 m/s (112 mph), the upthrust of the air will be equal in

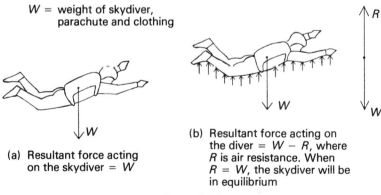

W = weight of skydiver,
   parachute and clothing

(a) Resultant force acting
   on the skydiver = W

(b) Resultant force acting on
   the diver = $W - R$, where
   R is air resistance. When
   $R = W$, the skydiver will be
   in equilibrium

Figure 2.24

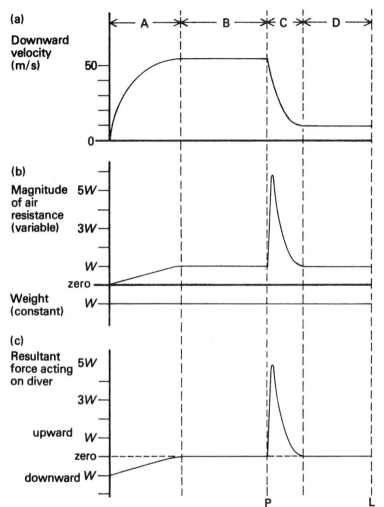

Figure 2.25 Variation in resultant force acting on a skydiver and his downward velocity during free fall and parachute landing.
A = period of acceleration after jumping out of aeroplane. Downward velocity increases to a maximum at which point the magnitude of $R = W$; B = period of free fall in equilibrium; P = parachute opens; C = period of deceleration; D = period of equilibrium prior to landing (L).

magnitude but opposite in direction to body weight. Consequently, the resultant force acting on the skydiver will be zero and provided that the orientation or shape of the body is not altered, the skydiver will continue to fall with a uniform downward velocity of about 50 m/s;

see Figure 2.24(b) and Figure 2.25(a) and (b). The skydiver will, therefore, be in a state of equilibrium. In order to land safely the skydiver must reduce downward velocity to about 10 m/s (22 mph). This is achieved by opening the parachute which suddenly presents a massive area to the air and greatly increases the air resistance. So great is the air resistance that for a very short time, about 2 seconds, the upward thrust of the air on the underside of the parachute is greater than the weight of the skydiver, i.e. $R > W$. Therefore, during this short period of time there will be a resultant upward force, $R - W$, acting on the skydiver; see Figure 2.25(b) and (c). Consequently the diver will experience a deceleration such that downward velocity will be rapidly reduced to around 10 m/s. As the skydiver decelerates the magnitude of the air resistance quickly drops to again equal that of body weight. A new state of equilibrium is thus obtained which continues until the skydiver lands on the ground. It is possible to estimate the average upward force acting on the diver during the short period of deceleration by applying Newton's Second Law of Motion,

$$\text{i.e.} \quad F = \frac{m(v - u)}{t}$$

where

F = average resultant force acting on the skydiver during the period of deceleration

m = mass of the skydiver, parachute and clothing

u = velocity of diver before opening parachute

v = velocity of diver after opening parachute

t = duration of period of deceleration

Since $m = 70$ kg, $u = 50$ m/s, $v = 10$ m/s and $t = 2$ s, then

$$F = \frac{70(10 - 50)}{2} = -1400 \text{ N}.$$

The negative sign indicates that F is a decelerating force and acts in an upward direction. F is the resultant of the two forces W and R acting on the skydiver. During the deceleration period, $R > W$, therefore,

$$F = R - W$$
$$\text{i.e.} \quad R = F + W$$
$$\text{since} \quad W = mg = 686 \text{ N},$$
$$R = 1400 + 686 = 2086 \text{ N}$$
$$= 212 \text{ kg wt}$$
$$\simeq 3W$$

This particular example shows that during the period of deceleration, air resistance exerts an average force of about three times body weight on the diver.

2.10.2 A man travelling in a lift

Whether the lift is at rest, moving upwards or downwards, there will be two forces acting on the man, i.e. the weight of his body, W, and the force, R, exerted by the floor of the lift on the man via his feet; see Figure 2.26. When the lift and, therefore, the man is at rest, $R = W$,

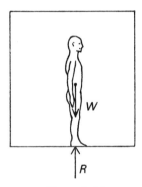

Figure 2.26

such that the resultant force acting on the man is zero. Consequently, the man will experience a force at his feet equal to his body weight. As the lift starts to move upwards, i.e. accelerate upwards from rest, there will be a resultant upward force acting on the man, i.e. $R > W$. Therefore, during the acceleration period, the man will feel heavier than normal since the force R acting on his feet will be *greater* than his body weight. At the end of the acceleration period, i.e. when the lift moves upwards with uniform velocity, the force R will again be equal to W so that the resultant force acting on the man will be zero. When the lift starts to slow down there will be a resultant downward force acting on the man, i.e. $W > R$. Therefore, during the deceleration period, i.e. as the upward velocity of the lift is reduced to zero, the man will feel lighter than normal since the force acting on his feet will be *less* than his body weight. As the lift starts to move downwards there will be a resultlant downward force acting on the man, i.e. $W > R$, such that he will feel lighter than normal. When the lift starts to slow down, i.e. as the downward velocity of the lift is reduced to zero, there will be a resultant upward force acting on the man, i.e. $R > W$, so that he

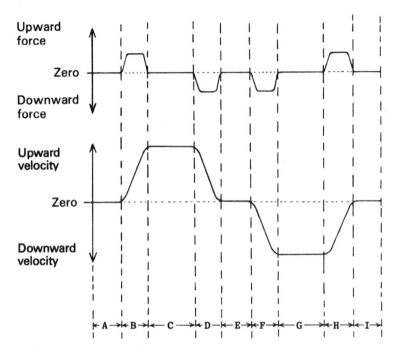

Figure 2.27 Relationship between resultant force acting on a man and his velocity when travelling in a lift.

A = lift at rest, $R = W$; resultant force on man = 0. B = Lift accelerating upwards, $R > W$; resultant upward force acting on man, i.e. he will feel heavier. C = Lift moving upwards with uniform velocity, $R = W$. D = Lift decelerating, $W > R$; resultant downward force acting on man, i.e. he will feel lighter. E = Lift at rest, $R = W$. F = Lift accelerating downwards, $W > R$. G = Lift moving downwards with uniform velocity, $R = W$. H = Lift decelerating, $R > W$. I = Lift at rest, $R = W$.

will feel heavier than normal. Figure 2.27 shows the relationship between the resultant force acting on the man and his velocity as the lift moves upwards and downwards from rest. The reader can easily verify these observations by travelling in a lift while standing on a set of bathroom scales. The amount by which a person feels heavier or lighter when travelling in a lift can be estimated by considering the acceleration of the lift. For example, consider a man of 70 kg wt travelling in a lift which accelerates upwards at $0.6 \, \text{m/s}^2$. There will be a resultant upward force of $R - W$ acting on the man. From Newton's second law,

$$R - W = ma$$

where

$$m = \text{mass of man} = 70\,\text{kg}$$
$$a = \text{upward acceleration} = 0.6\,\text{m/s}^2$$
$$W = 70\,\text{kg wt} = 686\,\text{N}$$

i.e.
$$R = ma + W$$
$$= (70 \times 0.6) + 686\,\text{N}$$
$$= 728\,\text{N} = 1.06\,W$$

Therefore, during the acceleration period, the man would feel heavier than normal by about 4 kg wt. The greater the upward acceleration of the lift the heavier the man would feel. For example, when a rocket lifts off from its launching pad the acceleration is so great that the upward force exerted on an astronaut inside the rocket is many times the weight of the astronaut, i.e. he feels many times heavier than normal. If the lift in the above example accelerates downwards at $0.6\,\text{m/s}^2$ there will be a resultant downward force of $W - R$ acting on the man. From Newton's Second Law,

$$W - R = ma$$

i.e.
$$R = W - ma$$
$$= 686 - (70 \times 0.6)\,\text{N}$$
$$= 644\,\text{N} = 0.94\,W$$

i.e. during the period of downward acceleration of the lift, the man would feel lighter by about 4 kg wt. The greater the downward acceleration of the lift, the lighter the man would feel.

2.11 Newton's Third Law of Motion

When a soccer player kicks a ball, there is a period of time in which the ball and the player's boot are in contact. During this time force is applied to the ball (the action force). Simultaneously, the player will be aware of a force pushing against his or her foot (the reaction force); see Figure 2.28. Furthermore, the harder the player kicks the ball, i.e. the greater the action force, the greater will be the reaction force experienced pushing against the foot. Similarly, the more force a shot putter applies to the shot the greater will be the reaction force pushing against the shot putter's hand; see Figure 2.29. These examples show that whenever one object, A, exerts a force on another object, B, then B will exert a force on A. What is not so evident, however, is that the forces are equal in magnitude as well as opposite in direction. This phenomenon is the basis of Newton's Third Law of Motion. The law,

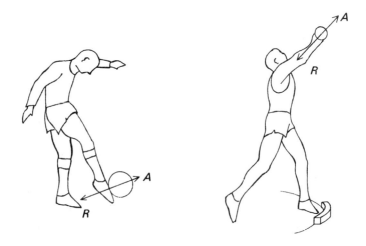

Figure 2.28   **Figure 2.29**

sometimes referred to as the law of interaction, may be expressed as follows:

> *Whenever one object exerts a force on another, there will be an equal and opposite force exerted by the second object on the first.*

Alternatively, *to every action there is an equal and opposite reaction.* Consider the force exerted by and, therefore, on the head of a soccer player when heading the ball.

If F = average force exerted on the ball,

u = 20 m/s = velocity of the ball as it comes into contact with the player's head

v = 15 m/s = velocity of the ball as it leaves the player's head.

Assume u and v are in opposite directions.

m = 0.4 kg = mass of the ball

t = 0.05 s = time the ball is in contact with the player's head.

From Newton's Second Law of Motion,

$$F = \frac{m(v - u)}{t}$$

Since u is in the opposite direction to F, it is given a negative sign in the calculation of F; i.e.,

$$F = \frac{0.4(15 - (-20))}{0.05}$$

$$= 280\,\text{N} = 28.5\,\text{kg wt}$$

The values of u, v, m and t used in the above example are fairly typical of those which occur during the game. The force acting on the head may be considerably greater than 28.5 kg wt, especially when the ball is heavy and/or travelling very quickly. Considering that some players, particularly those who play in defensive positions, may be required to head the ball many times during a game, it is hardly surprising that they sometimes suffer from concussion during or after a game.

There are many occasions when it is necessary to reduce the magnitude of forces acting on the human body in order to prevent injury. Such occasions occur largely during the performance of two types of movement:

(i) Stopping a moving object, e.g. catching a cricket ball, trapping a soccer ball on the chest, riding a punch in boxing.

(ii) Stopping the human body, e.g. landing from a height, falling, as in judo, wrestling and skateboarding.

The purpose of these movements is to reduce the momentum of the human body or that of a moving object to zero. In doing so, the deceleration force, as in landing from a height, or the reaction to the decelerating force, as in catching a cricket ball, will be exerted on the body tissues, i.e. the muscles, ligaments and bones. If the rate of change of momentum of the moving object is very high, i.e. if the decelerating force applied to the object is very large, the body tissues may not be able to withstand such a force and injury may occur. From Newton's Second Law of Motion the greater the length of time in which the momentum of a moving object is dissipated, the smaller will be the force required to bring the object to rest, and consequently the less chance of damage occurring to the object and the stopping agent. This principle is applied to good effect in many sports which involve one of the types of movement listed above. The essential features of each type of movement will now be described with reference to specific examples.

2.11.1 Stopping an object

Consider the act of catching a cricket ball. If an attempt is made to catch the ball with the arms and hands held fairly rigidly in readiness for the catch, the ball will tend to decelerate very quickly on impact with the hands, such that the fingers may not have time to flex around the ball and it will tend to bounce out of the hands. At the same time, the reaction to the high force exerted by the hands on the ball may injure the hands. However, if the arms and hands are held fairly loosely prior to the catch, i.e. with the wrists slightly extended and the elbows and fingers slightly flexed, the impact of the ball on the hands will tend to flex the elbows, rather like compressing a spring, such that the hands move with the ball towards the chest; see Figure 2.30. The movement

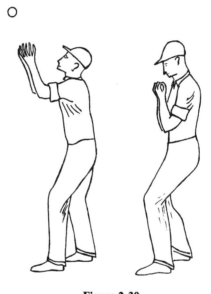

Figure 2.30

of the hands in the direction of the decelerating ball allows the fingers sufficient time to flex around the ball, and since the momentum of the ball is dissipated over a longer time the average force exerted by the hands on the ball and, therefore, the reaction force exerted on the hands is considerably reduced. The deceleration period of the ball can be lengthened even further and the force acting on it reduced even further by moving the trunk in the direction of the ball, i.e. downwards and/or backwards. A slip fielder may be seen to fall or roll backwards in the process of taking a catch, especially when the ball is moving very quickly. Trapping a soccer ball on the chest is a similar action to catching. As the ball contacts the chest the trunk is moved backwards thereby dissipating the momentum of the ball over a longer period of time and reducing the force exerted on the ball and chest to a minimum, with the result that the ball drops at the feet of the player instead of bouncing away.

2.11.2 Stopping the human body

(A) LANDING FROM A VERTICAL FALL

Upon striking the floor the longer the period of deceleration, the smaller will be the average force acting on the body during landing and, therefore, the less chance of injury. When landing on the feet it is advisable to contact the floor as soon as possible, i.e. with the legs fully extended; see Figure 2.31(a). This will maximise the period of deceleration and minimise the force acting on the body as the ankle, knee and hip joints move from a position of full extension to one of full flexion; see Figure 2.31(b). In doing so, the extensor muscles of the ankle, knee and hip joints 'absorb' the force of landing by stretching (eccentric contractions) and dissipate the force as heat within the muscles. The same principle applies when landing on the hands. Consider the force acting

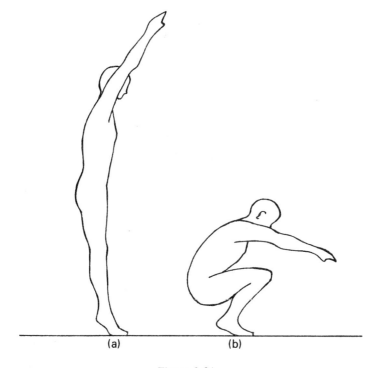

(a)   (b)

Figure 2.31

on the body when landing on the feet from a vertical fall, as in Figure
2.31. During the landing period the body exerts a force against the floor
and consequently experiences an equal and opposite force called the
ground reaction force. Therefore, during the landing period the body
is acted upon by two forces, i.e. the weight of the body, W, acting vertically downwards and the ground reaction force, R, acting vertically
upwards; see Figure 2.32. It is the resultant upward force of $R - W$

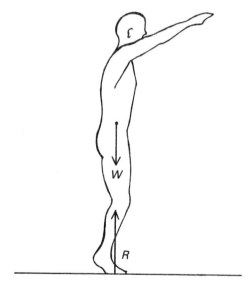

Figure 2.32

which is responsible for decelerating the body during the landing
period. The ground reaction force first of all increases then decreases
until it is equal in magnitude to body weight. The body will then be at
rest since the resultant of R and W will be zero. If a man falls through
a distance of 1 m, which may occur after a vault or tumbling movement
in gymnastics, the velocity of his body when he contacts the floor will
be approximately 4.4 m/s. If he lands very heavily, i.e. without bending
his legs very much, the period of deceleration will be rapid, i.e. about
0.1 s. From Newton's Second Law,

$$R - W = \frac{m(v - u)}{t}$$

where

$$m \ = \ \text{mass of man} \ = \ 70\,\text{kg}$$
$$u \ = \ 4.4\,\text{m/s}$$
$$v \ = \ 0$$
$$t \ = \ 0.1\,\text{s}$$

since u is in the opposite direction to the resultant upward force $R - W$ it is given a negative sign in the calculation; i.e.,

$$R - W \ = \ \frac{70(0 - (-4.4))}{0.1} \ = \ 3080\,\text{N}$$

since $W = 70\,\text{kg wt} = 686\,\text{N}$

$$R - 686\,\text{N} \ = \ 3080\,\text{N}$$
$$\text{i.e.} \quad R \ = \ 3766\,\text{N}$$
$$\simeq \ 5.5\,W$$

The calculated value of R, five and a half times body weight, is the average force acting directly on the feet during the landing period. The peak value of R would be greater than $5\frac{1}{2}\,W$ and could quite easily result in serious injury to the feet. If the man fully flexes his legs on landing the deceleration period could be increased to approximately 0.4 s and the average force exerted on the feet considerably reduced; i.e.,

$$R - W \ = \ \frac{70(0 - (-4.4))}{0.4} \ = \ 770\,\text{N}$$
$$R \ = \ 770 + 686 \ = \ 1456\,\text{N}$$
$$\simeq \ 2\,W$$

In some sports, such as gymnastics and judo, mats are used to decrease the forces on the body due to landing and thereby help to prevent injury. In athletics the heights achieved by high jumpers and especially pole vaulters necessitate very deep landing areas. In sports which involve a lot of jumping and landing – for example, basketball and volleyball – the players usually wear fairly thick-soled shoes and thick stockings in order to reduce the stress on the muscles, ligaments and bones of the feet and lower legs.

(B) FALLING BACKWARDS OR FORWARDS

In some sports, such as judo, wrestling and skateboarding, it is not always possible to land on the feet. In such instances it is advisable to maximise the area of body contact with the floor in order to spread the force of landing over as wide an area as possible and thereby reduce the force exerted on any single body part. This manoeuvre is sometimes referred to as the 'sit down and roll' principle. At the same time, the fleshy parts of the body – i.e. shoulders, upper arms, buttocks and thighs – should be used as striking surfaces as much as possible in order to protect the delicate and/or bony projections of the body, i.e. the head, elbows and knees. To this end skateboarders wear helmets, elbow pads and knee pads. Volleyball players and sometimes soccer goalkeepers also wear knee pads. Special clothing is worn by players in many sports in order to protect them from injury which would otherwise occur as a result of impact forces. In cricket, for example, a batsman wears gloves which are thickly padded on the outside. If he happens to be struck by the ball on the hand, most if not all of the momentum of the ball will be absorbed by compressing the glove material which is usually some form of sponge rubber. A batsman also wears leg pads for the same reason of protection. A wicket-keeper wears gloves not only for protection but also to increase the chance of a successful catch by increasing the catching area. In the days of prize fighting when the contestants fought without gloves the injuries sustained to head, body and hands were often very serious. In modern professional boxing the boxers wear gloves of a prescribed weight and structure which reduces the amount of force exerted between hand and body and consequently greatly reduces the chances of serious injury. During training, boxers usually wear head guards and fairly thick gloves as an added protection against head injury. In a number of sports, including mountaineering, canoeing, motor cycling and motor racing, the participants wear helmets to reduce the chances of head injury.

2.12 Pressure

When a man is standing upright on both feet the weight of his body is transmitted to the floor by the soles of his feet, i.e. the whole of the supporting area of his feet; see Figure 2.33. The supporting area of the feet will experience a force, i.e. the ground reaction force, equal and opposite to the weight of the man. The ground reaction force does not pass through a single point but is distributed over the supporting area of the feet. The force transmitted per unit area is referred to as the *pressure* on the supporting area. The supporting area of the feet of an adult male is approximately 200 square cm (cm^2). For a man weighing

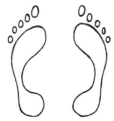

Figure 2.33 Supporting area of the feet

70 kg wt the average pressure on the supporting area of his feet is given by,

$$\text{Pressure} \quad = \quad \frac{\text{force}}{\text{area}} \quad = \quad \frac{70}{200} \quad = \quad 0.35\,\text{kg wt/cm}^2$$
$$= \quad 5\,\text{lb wt/in}^2$$

If the man lies down on his back, the weight of his body will be supported by a much larger area which will include parts of the upper back, the buttocks, the elbows, the calves and the heels. The pressure on this larger area, which is about 1200 cm², is given by,

$$\frac{70}{1200} \quad = \quad 0.06\,\text{kg wt/cm}^2 \quad = \quad 0.8\,\text{lb wt/in}^2$$

It should be evident that the larger the area supporting a particular weight the smaller will be the pressure on that area. In some sports – for example, wrestling, judo and skateboarding – the damage to the body resulting from a fall is minimised by maximising the area of body contact with the floor, i.e. 'the sit down and roll' principle. In a number of sports the players fix studs or spikes to the soles of their shoes to increase the grip or friction between themselves and the playing surface. Figure 2.34(a) shows one of the boots of a soccer player where the studs sink fully into the pitch such that the weight of the body is transmitted directly to the playing surface by the soles of the boots; see Figure 2.34(b). When playing on a fairly hard surface the studs may not sink fully into the pitch such that the weight of the body is transmitted indirectly by the soles of the boots and directly by the studs. The ground reaction force will, therefore, be exerted via the studs which constitute a very small area in comparison with the soles of the boots. This results in an increase in the pressure on those parts of the feet directly above the studs; see Figure 2.34(c) and (d). The actual pressure on any part of the foot will depend upon the rigidity of the sole of the boot; the

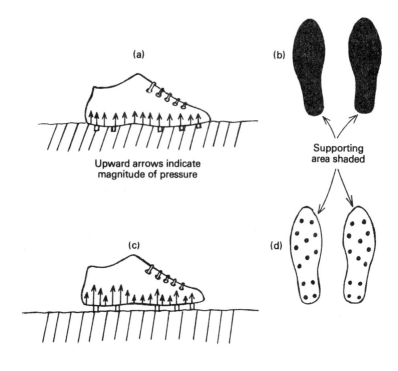

Figure 2.34

stiffer the sole, the more evenly distributed will be the pressure on the foot; see Figure 2.35(a). In contrast, if the sole is fairly pliable, the distribution of the upward force exerted by each stud will be slight such that the pressure on those parts of the foot directly above the studs will be considerably greater than the pressure on other parts of the sole of the foot; see Figure 2.35(b). To illustrate this point let us assume that there is no distribution of the upward forces exerted by the studs, such that the ground reaction force is shared only by those parts of the soles of the boots in contact with the studs. On a moulded sole soccer boot there are usually 13 studs. The area of each stud is approximately 1 cm^2 such that the supporting area of both boots is approximately 26 cm^2. If the weight of the player is 70 kg wt, the pressure on those parts of the feet directly above the studs is given by,

$$\frac{70 \text{ kg wt}}{26 \text{ cm}^2} \quad = \quad 2.7 \text{ kg wt/cm}^2 \quad = \quad 40 \text{ lb wt/in}^2$$

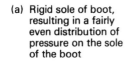

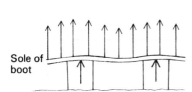

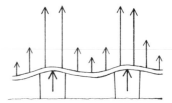

Reaction forces exerted
by studs on sole of boot

Figure 2.35

This hypothetical figure suggests an eight-fold increase in the pressure on certain parts of the feet in comparison with when the ground reaction force is evenly distributed. However, the upward forces exerted by the studs will always be at least partially distributed. Nevertheless, the example does indicate that when body weight is supported by the studs alone the pressure on certain parts of the foot is increased considerably even when standing. Any kind of propulsive movement of the legs will increase this pressure even more. As the pressure increases so does the possibility of damage to the soft tissues of the under-surface of the foot, particularly the heel and ball.

Boots with fairly rigid soles will seriously impair the natural movement of the feet and probably result in blisters, callouses and other more serious injuries. Bearing in mind that the larger the supporting area the lower the pressure, it is vitally important to choose studs which will allow the maximum area of contact between the soles of the boots and the playing surface. As a general rule, the harder the playing surface the shorter the studs should be. On a frozen or bone-dry pitch, flat-soled boots should be worn. These will minimise the possibility of soft-tissue damage due to pressure and provide the necessary friction between boots and playing surface.

2.13 Friction
Whenever one object moves or tends to move across the surface of another there will be a force parallel to the surfaces in contact which will oppose the movement or tendency to move. This force is called friction. Consider a block of wood resting on a level table. The only

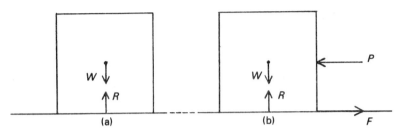

Figure 2.36

forces acting on the block of wood are the weight of the block, W, which is transmitted to the table and the reaction force, R, exerted by the table on the block; see Figure 2.36(a). If an attempt is made to move the block along the surface of the table by pushing against the side of the block, the frictional force, F, will begin to operate and oppose the tendency of the block to move; see Figure 2.36(b). Until the block begins to move the frictional force will exactly equal the horizontal force, P, pushing against the side of the block. The frictional force, therefore, has a maximum value which is proportional to:

  (i) The degree of roughness of the two surfaces in contact.
  (ii) The reaction force R.

The three variables are related by the equation,

$$F = \mu R \tag{1}$$

where μ (Greek letter mu) is a measure of the roughness of the surfaces in contact and is called the coefficient of friction between the surfaces. The magnitude of μ depends upon the nature of the two surfaces in contact; for example, it is about 0.3–0.5 for wood on wood and 0.1–0.6 for wood on metal. When $\mu = 0$, the surfaces in contact will be perfectly smooth or frictionless. For any two objects in contact, μ will be slightly less when the objects are sliding on each other than when the objects are at rest but tending to slide on each other. Consequently, for any two surfaces in contact there is a coefficient of sliding (dynamic) friction, μ_S, and a coefficient of limiting (static) friction, μ_L. This phenomenon can be demonstrated by a simple experiment. Place a block of wood weighing about 1 kg wt on a level polished wooden table. Apply a horizontal force to the block *very* gradually and note the maximum force recorded on the spring balance before the block just begins to move. The coefficient of limiting friction between the block and the table can then be estimated as follows,

$$\mu_L = \frac{F_1}{R}$$

where F_1 is the maximum force recorded on the spring balance and R is the weight of the block. Repeat the experiment and observe the decrease in force as the block begins to move. Note the force F_2 required to move the block slowly but steadily along the surface of the table. F_2 will be less than F_1 such that μ_S will be less than μ_L:

$$\mu_S = \frac{F_2}{R}$$

Results similar to those in row 1 of Table 2.4 will be obtained. This simple experiment demonstrates the general principle that the maximum amount of friction which opposes movement when one object slides on another, i.e. sliding friction, is less than the frictional force which opposes the tendency of the object to start to slide on the other, i.e. limiting friction. It is easier, therefore, to keep an object sliding than it is to start the object sliding. For example, pushing a sledge, pushing or pulling a box across the floor.

Table 2.4 Weight of block of wood = 1.1 kg wt

Supporting surface	Limiting friction		Sliding friction	
	F(kg wt)	μ_L	F(kg wt)	μ_S
Polished wooden table	0.55	0.5	0.23	0.21
Formica	0.33	0.3	0.18	0.16
Resin floor tile	0.8	0.7	0.38	0.34
Plain rubber mat	0.9	0.8	0.45	0.41

Different materials have different coefficients of friction and this can be demonstrated by varying the nature of the supporting surface in the experiment described above. Rows 2, 3 and 4 of Table 2.4 show the results obtained for μ_L and μ_S between the block of wood and three other supporting surfaces. From equation (1), the frictional force, limiting or sliding, exerted between two surfaces is independent of the area of contact between the adjoined surfaces. This can be demonstrated by turning the block of wood on its side, i.e. creating a smaller or larger area of contact with the supporting surface, and measuring μ_L or μ_S. Whatever the area in contact between two materials, μ_L and μ_S will always be the same.

In many games and sports it is necessary for the participants to create a certain amount of friction between their feet and the playing surface or between their hands and some implement such as a club, racket or pole, in order to prevent slipping. In such cases the frictional force is increased by increasing μ_L and, therefore, μ_S between the contacting surfaces. This is achieved by 'roughening' either or both of the contacting surfaces or by interposing some substance between the contacting surfaces. Mountaineers, cricketers, golfers and track athletes, for example, fix spikes to the soles of their shoes; soccer and rugby players use studs. Participants in other sports such as basketball, volleyball, squash and badminton wear shoes which have soles specially designed to increase the grip between shoes and playing surface. It follows that for most indoor sports the playing surface should not be highly polished since this will reduce the coefficient of friction between shoes and playing surface and, therefore, increase the possibility of slipping. A word of caution, however, since on occasions too much friction between shoes and playing surface will tend to impair skilful movement and may result in injury if the player turns very sharply. In such an instance, the foot should ideally turn with the body. However, the friction between shoe and playing surface will oppose the turning movement of the foot. Too much friction will prevent the foot turning at all so that the leg is twisted on the foot which may result in damage to the tissues of the knee joint, lower leg and ankle joint. Any soccer or rugby player whose studs are too long is particularly prone to this type of injury.

There are many non-sporting situations in which the creation of an adequate amount of friction is important; for example, an injured or aged person walking with the aid of crutches or a stick relies very much for his or her safety on the friction developed between the ends of the crutches and the floor. For this reason, rubber tips are usually fixed to the ends of the crutches since rubber has a very high coefficient of friction with almost any other material.

In some activities, skilful performance depends upon reducing the friction between shoes and floor to a certain extent. In ballroom dancing, for example, good technique necessitates that the dancer can slide and turn on the floor with as little resistance as possible. Consequently, not only is the floor highly polished but so are the soles of the dancer's shoes. Similarly, top-class skiers wax the underside of their skis to reduce the amount of friction between the skis and the snow to an absolute minimum.

So far the role of friction as an external force acting on an object, i.e. between the surfaces of two adjacent objects, has been discussed. To prevent slipping adequate friction must be developed between the adjacent surfaces, i.e. in order to turn a door knob or a steering wheel, to pull on a rope or grip a tennis racket, friction must be developed between the surfaces of the hand and the other object. Within the human body, however, friction between the various body tissues must be eliminated as much as possible in order to reduce the likelihood of damage and/or wear. The human body is made up of a number of different tissues which lie adjacent to each other. Even the slightest movement involves a certain amount of sliding of the various tissues on each other. Unless the adjacent surfaces are adequately lubricated, frictional forces will operate when sliding occurs. Whenever friction develops a certain amount of heat is generated. Too much friction and/or heat will tend to damage and/or wear the body tissues. In machines, parts which slide on each other are usually highly polished and friction is reduced even more by lubricating the sliding surfaces with oil or grease. Similar mechanisms exist within the human body. All of the freely moveable joints of the body are lined by a synovial membrane which produces synovial fluid. The latter is a transparent viscous fluid, resembling the white of an egg, which serves to lubricate the articulating surfaces of joints. The articulating surfaces are normally extremely smooth so that in association with the synovial fluid they produce a system five times as slippery as ice on ice. Consequently, the amount of friction, if any, developed between the articulating surfaces during joint movement is extremely small. When the synovial membrane is damaged, which may result from a hard blow on a joint, it produces large amounts of fluid which causes the joint to swell. With rest the excess fluid is gradually absorbed. However, severe damage or disease of the synovial membrane may impair its fluid-producing function such that fluid of insufficient viscosity is produced. The latter will result in an increase in the amount of friction produced during joint movement with the possibility of damage, i.e. roughening of the articular surfaces.

The lubricating function of synovial fluid is particularly important in the major weight-bearing joints of the body, i.e. the hips, knees and ankles. The articulating surfaces of these joints are under considerable pressure even when the individual is standing upright and any kind of propulsive movement of the legs will increase this pressure even more. The greater the pressure, the greater the potential frictional force between the articulating surfaces. It is vital, therefore, that any kind of injury to these joints, especially the knee joints, should be treated promptly so that the normal lubricating function of the synovial membrane is restored as soon as possible and damage to the articulating surfaces minimised. For example, in a normal knee joint the movements of flexion and extension involve a sliding–rolling action between the articulating surfaces of the femoral and tibial condyles. The removal of a meniscus, however, frequently results in an excessive amount of sliding between the articulating surfaces. If this condition is associated with an impaired synovial membrane there is a considerable possibility of permanent damage to the articulating surfaces. Wearing of articulating surfaces is similar to the wearing of brake pads in the wheels of a motor car. When braking occurs, an enormous amount of friction and, therefore, heat is generated between brake pad and wheel. Consequently the brake pads gradually wear out and eventually have to be replaced.

Apart from in joints, synovial membranes are present in other parts of the body where different tissues slide over each other. For example, most of the tendons of the muscles which flex and extend the wrist, fingers, ankles and toes pass over, through or around bones and ligaments. To reduce friction between tendon and bone or between tendon and ligament the tendons are enclosed within synovial sheaths. A synovial sheath is an elongated, closed sac which forms a sleeve around the tendon. Aggravation of the synovial sheaths resulting from unaccustomed overuse of the various muscles leads to a condition known as tenosynovitis. Squash players are particularly prone to this type of injury to the flexor and extensor tendons of the wrist. A synovial bursa is a flattened sac interposed between two surfaces that slide on each other and which prevents friction. Bursae are located most frequently between the deeper layers of the skin and underlying bone (subcutaneous bursae) and between individual muscles (submuscular bursae). For example, there is a large bursa between the skin and the patella. Aggravation of this bursa leads to a condition known as prepatellar bursitis or housemaid's knee. Excessive and/or repetitive movement of the shoulder joint in activities such as swimming or javelin throwing may aggravate the bursa between the deltoid and supraspinatus muscles giving rise to a condition known as subacromial bursitis.

A blister is a form of bursa which occurs in response to unaccustomed friction on certain parts of the skin, especially the hands and feet. A blister is a short-term safety mechanism which protects the deep layers of the skin from sustained and/or excessive friction resulting from relatively infrequent experiences such as stiff shoes rubbing against the feet or the handle of a screwdriver rubbing against the hand. The body responds to such friction by producing a layer of fluid between the superficial and deep layers of the skin, thereby protecting the deep layers from further damage. A blister is usually painful, which is the body's way of asking for the cause of the irritation to be removed so that no further damage may occur. In the long term, the body will respond to sustained friction on a particular part of the skin by thickening the superficial layer of the skin. For example, in comparison with other parts of the body, the skin on the heel and ball of each foot is subjected to fairly sustained pressure and/or frictional force. Not surprisingly, therefore, the skin on the heel and ball of each foot is much thicker than at any other part of the body except, perhaps, for the palmer surface of the hands of a manual worker.

2.14   Ground reaction

Consider a man standing upright as in Figure 2.37(a). The only forces acting on the man are his body weight, W, and the ground reaction force, R, which is equal and opposite to W such that the resultant force acting on the man is zero. Since W is constant the only way the man can move his body up or down is to increase or decrease R, thereby creating a resultant upward $(R - W)$ or downward $(W - R)$ force, respectively.

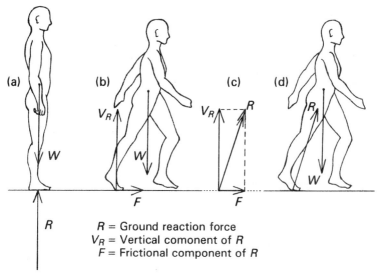

R = Ground reaction force
V_R = Vertical comonent of R
F = Frictional component of R

Figure 2.37

In order to move horizontally – i.e. forwards, backwards or sideways – the man, as shown in Figure 2.37(a), must be able to create an external force which acts on his body in the direction he wants to move, i.e. if he wants to move forward there must be a forward directed external force acting on his body. The only object capable of providing an external force on the man is the earth. Therefore, in order to move forward the man pushes backwards against the earth with his foot. Provided that his foot does not slip backwards, i.e. provided frictional force can be developed between his foot and the floor, it follows from Newton's Third Law of Motion that the man will experience at his foot a force, F, equal in magnitude but opposite in direction to that which he applies against the floor; see Figure 2.37(b). However, the frictional force, F, does not move the body forwards; it prevents the foot slipping backwards so that the leg can extend against a fixed point, thereby moving the body forwards; see Figure 2.38. The greater the

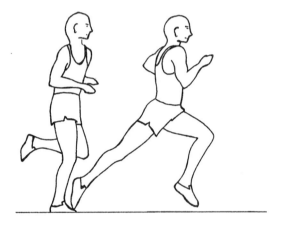

Figure 2.38

frictional force, the more rapidly the body will move forward. Any frictional force will prevent or oppose movement between two adjoined surfaces but it never initiates movement. If the man in Figure 2.37(a) could not develop frictional force between his feet and the floor he would not be able to move horizontally; he could jump off the floor vertically, but until a non-vertical force acted on him – i.e. any force with a horizontal component – the line of action of his body weight would remain over the same spot on the floor.

The ground reaction force always has a vertical component which counteracts body weight, as shown in Figure 2.37(a). When the body moves horizontally (i.e., when the displacement of the body has a horizontal component) such as running along a level track or up the slope of a hill, the ground reaction will also have a frictional component; see Figure 2.37(b–d). The magnitude and direction of the ground reaction and, therefore, of V_R and F, will depend upon the type of activity. From a sprint start, for example, the athlete wants to generate maximum velocity forwards; consequently, the frictional component of the ground reaction will be relatively large; see figure 2.39(a). Starting blocks are normally used since they can be securely fixed to the track, thereby minimising the chance of the athlete's feet and the blocks slipping backwards as he or she drives out of the blocks. As the athlete accelerates up to maximum speed the frictional force will act in a forward direction, as in Figure 2.39(a). However, when he or she slows down at the end of a race the frictional force will act in the

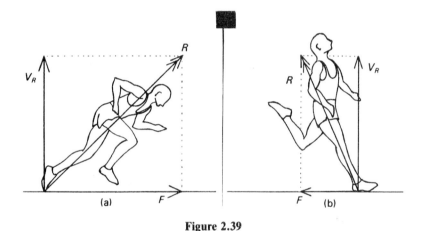

Figure 2.39

opposite direction since it is then a decelerating force; see Figure 2.39(b). The high jumper requires maximum vertical velocity at take-off such that during the take-off period the vertical component of the ground reaction will be very large in relation to the frictional component; see Figure 2.40(a). The vertical component must be large since it is not only responsible for counteracting body weight but also for generating the momentum necessary to lift the body off the ground. During take-off the magnitude of the vertical component is about three times body weight for a world-class high jumper. At take-off, the long jumper needs to project the body forwards and upwards with maximum velocity. He or she builds up forward linear momentum during the run-up so that during the take-off period effort can be concentrated on achieving height by pushing downwards rather than downwards and backwards. There will be a certain amount of frictional force but horizontal velocity will be almost entirely due to the speed of the run-up; see Figure 2.40(b).

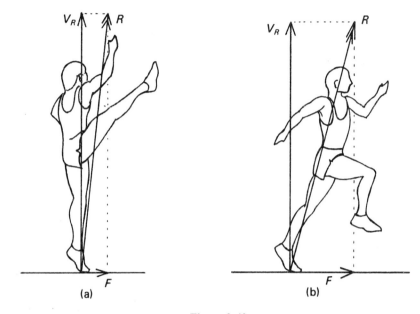

Figure 2.40

2.15 The importance of the free body diagram in the solution of mechanical problems

The student of elementary mechanics sometimes has difficulty in understanding the operation of Newton's Third Law of Motion. For example, consider a man pushing a large box across a level floor; see Figure 2.41. By Newton's Third Law, the force A exerted by the man on the box will be equal and opposite to the force R exerted by the box on the man. The question often asked is, 'If the force on the box is the

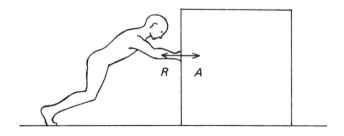

Figure 2.41

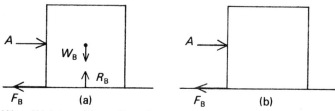

W_B = Weight of box; R_B = Ground reaction to weight of box;
F_B = Friction between box and floor.

Figure 2.42

same as that on the man's hands, how does the box move forwards?'
The misunderstanding results from not taking into consideration all of
the forces acting on the man and on the box. An object will move from
rest only when the resultant of *all* of the forces acting on the object is
greater than zero. To understand the nature of the resultant force acting
on an object it is necessary to consider all of the individual forces acting
on the object by means of a free body diagram. An understanding of
the free body diagram is the key to understanding mechanics. The
reader should draw clear and complete free body diagrams for every
mechanical problem he or she attempts to solve. When such a problem
involves two or more objects in contact with each other, a separate free
body diagram should be drawn for each object.

The forces acting on the box in the example referred to above are
represented in Figure 2.42(a). The only horizontal forces acting on the
box, i.e. the only forces which determine whether the box moves
horizontally across the floor, are A and F_B; see Figure 2.42(b). It
follows, therefore, that the box will move forward if,

$$A \ > \ F_B \tag{1}$$

The forces acting on the man are represented in Figure 2.43(a). The only
horizontal forces acting on the man are R and F_M; see Figure 2.43(b).
Whether the man is able to move the box forwards depends upon the
amount of friction which he can create at his feet. If he can create a
frictional force F_M at his feet which is greater than the resistance R of
the box, then the box will move forward, i.e. the box will move forward
if,

$$F_M > R$$

Since R is equal in magnitude to A, the box will move forward if,

$$F_M > A \tag{2}$$

Therefore, from equations (1) and (2) the box will move forward if $F_M > F_B$, i.e. if the friction developed between the man's feet and the floor is greater than the friction between the box and the floor.

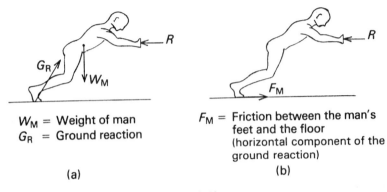

W_M = Weight of man
G_R = Ground reaction

(a)

F_M = Friction between the man's feet and the floor (horizontal component of the ground reaction)

(b)

Figure 2.43

3

Angular Motion

3.1 Centre of gravity

An object can be considered to consist of any number of separate pieces. Each piece will contribute a certain amount of weight to the total weight of the object. For example, in analysing human movement it is often beneficial to regard the body as a system of 14 separate segments; namely, the hands, the forearms, the upper arms, the head and neck, the trunk, the thighs, the lower legs, and the feet; see Figure 3.1(a). The total weight of the body, i.e. the resultant force

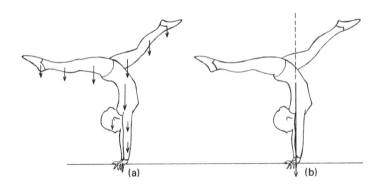

Figure 3.1

acting vertically downwards on the body, acts along a line called the line of action of body weight; see Figure 3.1(b). Consider Figure 3.2, which shows eight successive positions of a gymnast during the performance of a vault. As the gymnast moves through positions 2–7, the orientation of the different body parts to each other remains the same. The line of action of body weight is shown at each position.

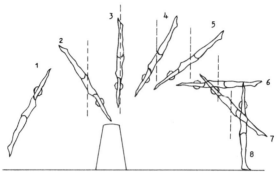

Figure 3.2

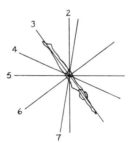

Figure 3.3

Figure 3.3 shows that when positions 3–7 are superimposed on position 2, the different lines of action of body weight intersect at a single point. This point is called the *centre of mass* or *centre of gravity* (c. of g.) of the gymnast with respect to the position under consideration. Any object behaves as if the whole of its weight is concentrated at its c. of g., i.e. as if the gravitational pull of the earth is exerted at the c. of g. For example, consider a book resting on a table as shown in Figure 3.4(a). The book can be gradually pushed over the edge of the

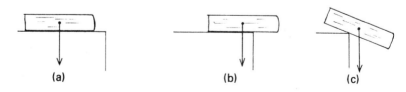

(a)   (b)   (c)

Figure 3.4

table but it will not fall until the c. of g. becomes unsupported, i.e. until the line of action of the weight of the book passes beyond the edge of the table; see Figure 3.4(b) and (c). The c. of g. of an object may be defined as the point at which the whole weight of the object can be considered to act. In a free body diagram, the tail of the vector representing the weight of an object begins at the c. of g. of the object.

The position of the c. of g. of an object depends upon the distribution of the weight of the object. For a regular shaped object such as a cube or oblong the c. of g. is situated at the geometric centre of the object; see Figure 3.5.

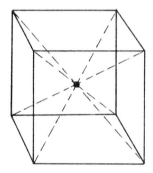

Figure 3.5

However, the c. of g. of an irregular shaped object, such as the human body, will be nearer the heavier end of the object. For example, when a man is standing upright the position of his c. of g. will be close to the level of his navel, i.e. about 54% of his stature when measured from the floor, and mid-way between the front and back of his body; see Figure 3.6(a). If he extends his arms in front of him as shown in Figure 3.6(b), his c. of g. will move slightly upwards and slightly forwards. By moving his arms from the position shown in Figure 3.6(b), to that shown in figure 3.6(c), his c. of g. will move slightly backwards and slightly upwards. Since the combined weight of both arms only comprise about 11% of total body weight, any movement of the arms results in only a slight change in the position of the c. of g. However, movement of larger segments results in relatively large changes in the position of the c. of g. For example, the trunk comprises about 50% of total body weight such that by bending forward, as shown in Figure 3.6(d), the c. of g. may move outside the body. During walking, running

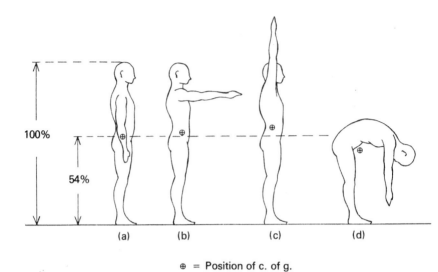

⊕ = Position of c. of g.
Figure 3.6

or any movement which involves continuous change in the orientation of the different body segments to each other, the position of the c. of g. will be continually changing although the amount of change may be slight.

3.2 Stability

Figure 3.7(a) and (b) represents a block of wood resting on a level surface with the face ABCD as its base of support. Since the supporting surface is horizontal the line of action of the weight of the block must intersect the base of support. If the block is tilted over on any of the edges AB, BC, CD, or AD and then released, it will return to its original position provided that at release the line of action of the weight of the block intersected the original base of support, as shown in Figure 3.7(c). However, if the line of action of the weight of the block does not intersect the original base of support, the block will not return to its original position when released but fall onto one of its other faces as shown in Figure 3.7(d) and (e).

With respect to a particular base of support, an object is said to be *stable* when the line of action of its weight intersects the base of support and *unstable* when it does not. In the above example, the block of wood is stable with respect to the base of support ABCD when in the position shown in Figure 3.7(c), and unstable when in the position shown in Figure 3.7(d).

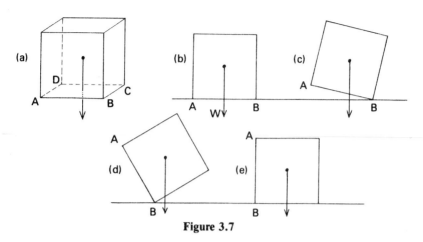

Figure 3.7

Consider a man standing upright as in Figure 3.8(a). For the man to remain in a balanced position, the line of action of his weight must remain within his base of support, i.e. the area of the floor beneath and between his feet as shown in figure 3.8(b). If the line of action of his weight passes outside this base of support he will fall over unless he establishes a new base of support. For example, if he leans forward from the position shown in Figure 3.8(a), such that the line of action of

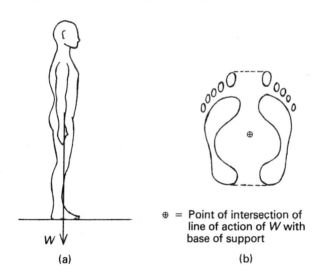

⊕ = Point of intersection of line of action of *W* with base of support

(a)   (b)

Figure 3.8

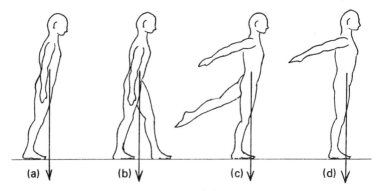

Figure 3.9

his weight moves in front of his base of support, he will fall over unless he moves one foot forward thereby bringing the line of action of his weight within a new base of support; see Figure 3.9(a) and (b). Alternatively, he may displace his c. of g. backwards by extending one leg and both arms backwards as shown in Figure 3.9(c) such that the line of action of his weight passes within the base of support provided by the grounded foot. If the degree of instability is slight, i.e. if the man perceives his unstable position quickly enough, he may be able to move his c. of g. back over the original base of support simply by extending both arms backwards as shown in Figure 3.9(d).

As the body moves from one position to another, one is not usually aware of the way in which the systems of the body responsible for balance automatically redistribute the body weight in order to maintain stability. For example, consider Figure 3.10(a) which shows a man

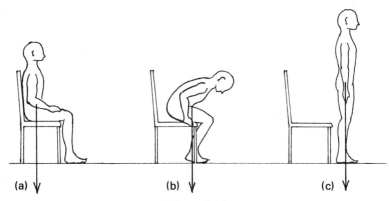

Figure 3.10

sitting on a chair. In order to stand up the man must move his c. of g. forwards by bending his trunk forwards and, perhaps, moving his feet backwards, so that the line of action of his weight passes from his base of support while sitting, the seat of the chair, to the base of support required for standing, the area of the floor beneath and between his feet (Figure 3.10(b)). He can then extend his legs and stand up (Figure 3.10(c)).

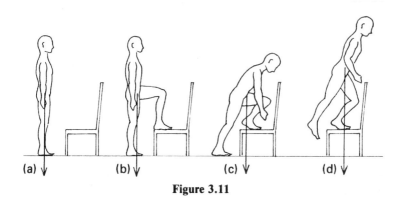

(a)   (b)   (c)   (d)

Figure 3.11

Figure 3.11 shows the movement of a man as he steps up onto a chair. He initiates the movement by putting one foot on the chair. In order to step up with the other foot he must move his c. of g. forwards so that the line of action of his weight passes within a new base of support provided by the foot of the leading leg. He can then extend the leading leg and stand up on the chair. Therefore, in walking up a flight of stairs, the c. of g. is continually shifted forwards over the leading foot.

When a man bends forward from a standing position as shown in Figure 3.12(a) and (b), his buttocks move backwards in relation to his feet in order to counterbalance his trunk, so that the line of action of his weight remains within his base of support. This can be easily demonstrated by asking the man to bend forward from a position of standing upright with his back and heels against a wall. Since his buttocks are prevented from moving backwards, the line of action of his weight soon passes in front of his base of support and he will fall over unless he moves one foot forward; see Figure 3.12(c) and (d).

It should be evident from the above example that the larger the base of support of an object, the more stable the object will be. However, the stability of an object depends not only on the size of its base of support but also on the height of its c. of g. above the base of support.

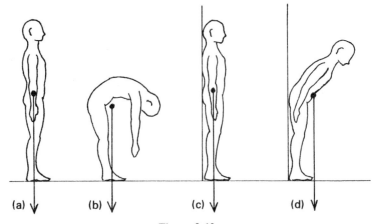

Figure 3.12

For example, consider two pieces of wood, 5 cm and 10 cm long, respectively, and both cut from the same piece of wood which has a square cross-section of 3 × 3 cm; see Figure 3.13. When the blocks rest

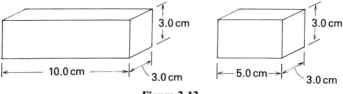

Figure 3.13

on any of their larger faces the c. of g. of one block will be at the same height as that of the other block, i.e. 1.5 cm above the base of support. If, from these positions, each block is tilted over on one of its end edges as shown in Figure 3.14, it will be observed that the block with the larger base of support must be tilted through an angle greater than 73° before it topples over. However, the block with the smaller base of support will topple over after being tilted through a much smaller angle.

If each block is stood on one of its smaller faces, the c. of g. of the larger block will be 5 cm above its base of support and that of the smaller block 2.5 cm above its base of support; see Figure 3.15(a) and (c). When the blocks are tilted from these positions it will be observed that the one with the higher c. of g. will topple over after being tilted

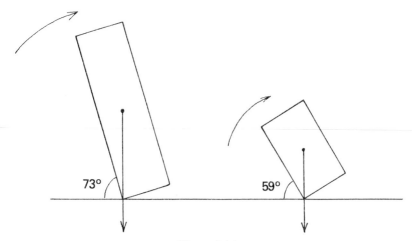

Figure 3.14

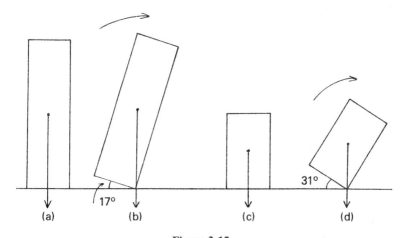

Figure 3.15

through a much smaller angle than that of the other block. The above experiments show that for a particular object, the larger the base of support and the lower the c. of g., the more stable the object will be. These principles are applied in many situations where the maintenance of stability is of prime importance. For example, a person recovering from a leg injury may use crutches or a walking stick in order to increase his or her base of support; see Figure 3.16(a) and (b).

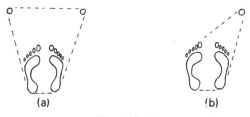

Figure 3.16

Motor vehicles, especially cars, tend to have a low c. of g. to reduce the possibility of the vehicle overturning. The 'prepared' stance of a wrestler or judo contestant is an example of the utilisation of both principles in that one foot is placed in front of the other, thereby creating a fairly large base of support and by slightly flexing the hips, knees and ankles the c. of g. of the contestant is lowered thereby further increasing his or her stability; see Figure 3.17.

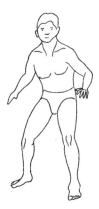

Figure 3.17

The smaller the base of support and the higher the c. of g. of an object the more difficult it will be for the object to remain in a stable position since greater control must be exerted over the shift of the c. of g. and, therefore, over the line of action of the weight of the object. For example, standing on one foot requires much greater control of the muscles of the grounded leg, especially those about the ankle joint, than is required of leg muscles when standing on two feet. In comparison

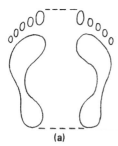 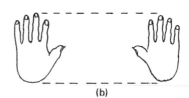

(a)　　　　　　　　　　　(b)

Figure 3.18

with standing on two feet, the base of support when standing on the hands is much wider and about two-thirds the length from front to back; see Figure 3.18. In addition, the height of the c. of g. in the handstand position is about the same as when standing on two feet. Theoretically, therefore, it should not be difficult to perform a handstand and certainly easier than standing on one foot. However, in order to perform a handstand considerable strength is required in the muscles which move the wrist and fingers, especially the finger flexors, and in the early stages of learning, the handstand is a very difficult balance to perform since the wrist and finger muscles are usually relatively weak. Standing on one hand is extremely difficult because of the small base of support and the considerable strength required in the wrist and finger muscles.

As the base of support of an object is gradually reduced in size, the amount of tolerance in the shift of the c. of g. of the object becomes progressively smaller if stability is to be maintained. Eventually the base of support becomes a knife edge or something close to it such as a tightrope or very narrow beam, whereupon the tolerance of c. of g. shift is zero; to remain in a stable position, the c. of g. of the object must stay directly above the line of support. Therefore, by balancing an object in a number of positions on a knife edge it should be possible to find the c. of g. of the object. For example, the position of the c. of g. of the human body may be estimated by balancing the body on a plane wooden board as shown in Figure 3.19(a). First of all it would be necessary to balance the board so that its c. of g. was located in the vertical plane through the line of support. The subject could then lie down on the board and move his or her body up and down the board until it balanced. The c. of g. of the body must then lie in the vertical plane through the line of support. By repeating the procedure in two other body positions, as shown for example in Figure 3.19(b) and (c), the position of the c. of g. of the body could be estimated by finding the point of intersection of the three planes.

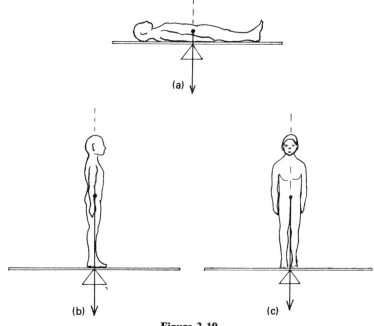

Figure 3.19

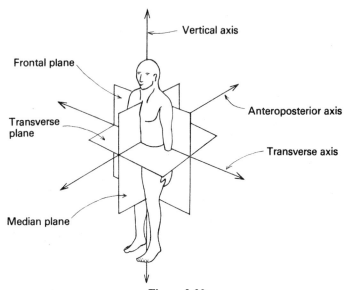

Figure 3.20

3.3 Planes and axes of reference

Angular or rotary motion always takes place about some specified straight line called an axis. In order to describe and analyse movements which involve rotation of either body parts or the whole body, it is useful to refer to certain axes *about* which and planes *in* which the rotation takes place. Three axes of reference are used to denote anteroposterior, transverse, and vertical directions with respect to the upright stance; see Figure 3.20. In describing the movement of a particular body part relative to the rest of the body, the axis of rotation of the body part is referred to as the 'local' axis of the body part. For example, flexion of the right arm takes place about its local transverse axis through the right shoulder joint; see Figure 3.21(a). Abduction of the left leg takes place about its local anteroposterior axis through the left hip joint; see Figure 3.21(b).

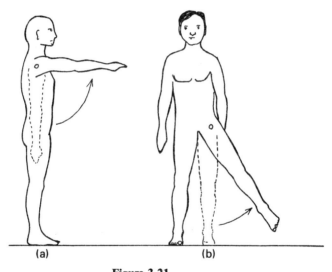

(a)   (b)

Figure 3.21

There are three principal planes of reference, two vertical and one horizontal. The median plane divides the body into right and left halves such that each is a virtual mirror image of the other; see Figure 3.20. A sagittal plane is any plane parallel to the median plane. The coronal or frontal plane, perpendicular to the median plane, divides the body into anterior and posterior portions. Any plane perpendicular to both the median and frontal planes is called a transverse plane. Figure 3.53 shows a gymnast performing a forward somersault. During the flight phase, he is seen to rotate in the median plane about a transverse axis through his c. of g.

3.4   Moment of a force

Consider a rectangular block of wood resting on a table, as shown in Figure 3.22(a). If the block is tilted over on one of its edges, as shown in Figure 3.22(b), the weight of the block will tend to turn the block about the supporting edge back to its original position. The tendency to restore the block to its original position is the result of the *moment* or *turning moment* of the weight of the block about the axis of rotation, i.e. the supporting edge B. The magnitude of the moment of the weight about edge B is equal to the product of the weight of the block and the perpendicular distance between the line of action of the weight and the axis of rotation (D).

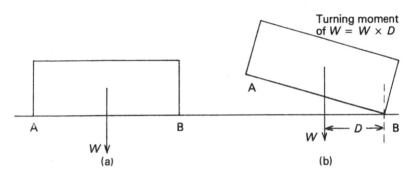

Figure 3.22

In general when a force acting on an object rotates or tends to rotate the object about some specific axis the turning moment of the force is defined as the product of the force and the perpendicular distance between the line of action of the force and the axis of rotation. The axis of rotation is often referred to as the *fulcrum*, and the perpendicular distance between the line of action of the force and the fulcrum is referred to as the *moment arm* of the force. The moment of a force is sometimes referred to as the *torque* of the force. For a given turning moment, the greater the force the smaller the moment arm and vice versa. For example, in trying to push open a heavy door much less force will be required if the force is applied to the side of the door furthest away from the hinges (i.e. a large moment arm) than if the force is applied to the door close to the hinges (i.e. a small moment arm); see Figure 3.23.

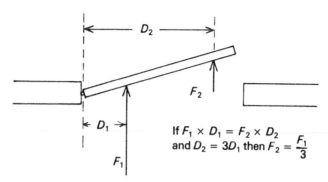

Figure 3.23

3.4.1 *Clockwise and anticlockwise moments*

When an object is acted upon by two or more forces which tend to rotate the object, the actual amount and speed of rotation which occurs will depend upon the resultant turning moment acting on the object, i.e. the resultant of all the individual turning moments. For example, consider two boys sitting on a seesaw as shown in Figure 3.24. If the seesaw is positioned such that its c. of g. is directly above the fulcrum,

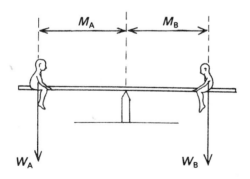

W_A = Weight of boy A
W_B = Weight of boy B
M_A = Moment arm of W_A
M_B = Moment arm of W_B

Figure 3.24

the weight of the seesaw will not have any turning moment about the fulcrum since its moment arm will be zero. Therefore, the only turning moments tending to rotate the seesaw will be those exerted by the two boys. Boy A will exert an anticlockwise turning moment of magnitude $W_A \times M_A$ and boy B will exert a clockwise turning moment of magnitude $W_B \times M_B$. When $W_A \times M_A$ is greater than $W_B \times M_B$, there will be a resultant anticlockwise moment acting on the seesaw such that boy B will be lifted upwards as boy A descends. When $W_A \times M_A$ is equal to $W_B \times M_B$, i.e. when the clockwise turning moment is equal to the anticlockwise turning moment, the resultant turning moment acting on the seesaw will be zero and the seesaw will not rotate in either direction. Consequently, if the weight of one of the boys was known it would be possible to find the weight of the other by first of all balancing the seesaw with one boy on each side of the fulcrum, both boys off the floor with the seesaw stationary, and then equating the clockwise and anticlockwise moments. For example, if $W_A = 40\,\text{kg wt}$ and in the balanced position $M_A = 1.5\,\text{m}$ and $M_B = 2.0\,\text{m}$, then by equating moments about the fulcrum,

$$\text{Anticlockwise moments (ACM)} = \text{Clockwise moments (CM)}$$

$$40\,\text{kg wt} \times 1.5\,\text{m} = W_B \times 2.0\,\text{m}$$

$$W_B = \frac{60\,\text{m}\,.\,\text{kg wt}}{2.0\,\text{m}}$$

$$W_B = 30\,\text{kg wt}$$

3.4.2   The position of the joint c. of g. of two weights

It was noted in Section 3.2 that to balance an object on a very narrow line of support it is necessary to position the object so that its c. of g. lies in the vertical plane through the line of support. Therefore, in the above example, when the seesaw is in a balanced positioned with both boys off the floor the c. of g. of the composite body consisting of seesaw plus boys must lie in the vertical plane through the fulcrum. However, since the seesaw was positioned with its c. of g. directly above the fulcrum, it follows that the joint c. of g. of the two boys, i.e. the point at which the combined weight of both boys can be considered to act, must also lie in the vertical plane through the fulcrum, otherwise the seesaw would rotate as the result of an unbalanced moment.

If boy A sat further away from the fulcrum such that $M_A = 2.25\,\text{m}$ and boy B moved further away from the fulcrum in order to balance the seesaw, M_B could be found by equating the clockwise and anti-clockwise moments as before; i.e.,

$$
\begin{aligned}
W_A &= 40 \text{ kg wt} \\
W_B &= 30 \text{ kg wt} \\
M_A &= 2.25 \text{ m}
\end{aligned}
$$

$$
\begin{aligned}
\text{ACM} &= \text{CM} \\
40 \text{ kg wt} \times 2.25 \text{ m} &= 30 \text{ kg wt} \times M_B \\
M_B &= 3.0 \text{ m}
\end{aligned}
$$

In each of the above examples, the seesaw was in a balanced position, i.e. the joint c. of g. of the two boys was directly above the fulcrum when,

$$
W_A \times M_A = W_B \times M_B
$$

$$
\frac{W_A}{W_B} = \frac{M_B}{M_A}
$$

Therefore, whatever the distance between the c. of g. of boy A and the c. of g. of boy B, $M_A + M_B$, the ratio of the moment arms of their weights about their joint c. of g., will remain constant. In the first example,

$$
\frac{M_B}{M_A} = \frac{2.0}{1.5} = 1.333
$$

In the second example,

$$
\frac{M_B}{M_A} = \frac{3.0}{2.25} = 1.333
$$

For any two weights, W_1 and W_2, the ratio of their moment arms, M_1 and M_2, about their joint c. of g. will be constant; i.e.,

$$
\frac{W_1}{W_2} = \frac{M_2}{M_1} = \text{a constant value} \tag{1}
$$

In the above examples, it was not necessary to involve the weight of the seesaw in the calculations since it had no moment about the fulcrum. However, provided that both the weight of the seesaw and the

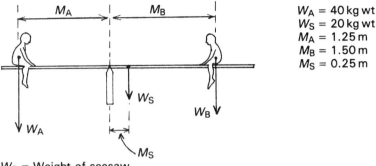

W_A = 40 kg wt
W_S = 20 kg wt
M_A = 1.25 m
M_B = 1.50 m
M_S = 0.25 m

W_S = Weight of seesaw
M_S = Moment of arm of W_S

Figure 3.25

position of its c. of g. are known, the weight of boy B could be found
by balancing the seesaw, with one boy on each side of the fulcrum,
about any point on its length and then equating clockwise and anticlockwise moments as before. For example, Figure 3.25 shows the
seesaw in a balanced position with the c. of g. of the seesaw to the right
of the fulcrum. By equating the anticlockwise and clockwise moments,

$$W_A \times M_A = (W_S \times M_S) + (W_B \times M_B)$$
$$40 \times 1.25 = (20 \times 0.25) + (1.5 \times W_B)$$
$$1.5\,W_B = 45$$
$$W_B = 30 \text{ kg wt}$$

In the above example the total clockwise moment was the sum of two
'component' moments, i.e. the moment of W_S and the moment of W_B.
The magnitude of the total clockwise moment could be exerted by a
single force equal to $W_S + W_B$ acting at the joint c. of g. of W_S and W_B.
To illustrate this principle, consider the position of the joint c. of g.
of W_S and W_B; see Figure 3.26.

From equation (1) $$\frac{W_S}{W_B} = \frac{M_{BG}}{M_{SG}}$$

Since $W_S = 20$ kg wt and $W_B = 30$ kg wt it follows that,

$$\frac{M_{BG}}{M_{SG}} = \frac{2}{3} \quad \text{and} \quad \frac{M_{BG}}{M_{BG} + M_{SG}} = \frac{2}{5}$$

Furthermore, since

$$M_{BG} + M_{SG} = M_B - M_S = 1.25 \text{ m}$$

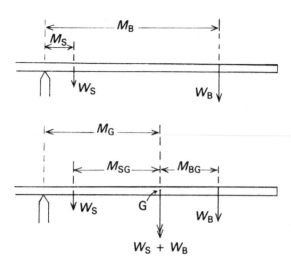

G = Position of joint c. of g. of W_S and W_B
M_{SG} = Moment arm of W_S about the joint c. of g. of W_S and W_B
M_{BG} = Moment arm of W_B about the joint c. of g. of W_S and W_B
M_G = Moment arm of joint c. of g. of W_S and W_B about the fulcrum

Figure 3.26

it follows that
$$\frac{M_{BG}}{1.25} = \frac{2}{5}$$

$$M_{BG} = 0.5\,\text{m}$$

$$M_{SB} = 0.75\,\text{m}$$

and
$$M_G = M_S + M_{SG} = 1.0\,\text{m}$$

Therefore, the joint moment of force of W_S and W_B is given by

$$(W_S + W_B) \times 1.0\,\text{m} = 50\,\text{m.kg wt}$$

But
$$(W_S \times M_S) + (W_B \times M_B) = 50\,\text{m.kg wt}$$

Therefore, the sum of the moments exerted by W_S and W_B is equivalent to the moment exerted by a single force of magnitude $W_S + W_B$ acting at the joint c. of g. of $W_S + W_B$. Irrespective of the number of forces exerting moments on an object, the sum of the moments is equivalent to the moment exerted by a single force equal in magnitude to the resultant of the individual forces acting at the joint c. of g. of the individual forces.

3.4.3 Two conditions for a state of equilibrium

It was noted in Section 2.10 that an object is in equilibrium when the resultant force acting on the object is zero. Consequently, in the above examples the sum of the weights of the two boys and the seesaw, the resultant downward force, must be counteracted by an equal and opposite force since the composite body consisting of seesaw plus boys is in equilibrium. This equal and opposite force R is exerted by the fulcrum on the seesaw. Figure 3.27(a) and (b) show the complete free body diagrams for the seesaw in the positions shown in Figures 3.24 and 3.25, respectively.

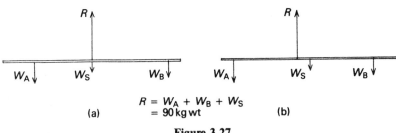

$$R = W_A + W_B + W_S$$
$$= 90 \, \text{kg wt}$$

(a) (b)

Figure 3.27

When an object is in equilibrium the resultant force acting on the object is zero. There is, however, one other condition which must prevail for an object to be in a state of equilibrium. The second condition, which was demonstrated in the above examples, is that the sum of the clockwise moments acting on an object must be equal to the sum of the anticlockwise moments. Furthermore, if an object is in equilibrium, the sum of the clockwise moments acting on the object will be equal to the sum of the anticlockwise moments with respect to *any point* (reference axis of rotation), within or outside the object. For example, consider the forces acting on the seesaw as shown in Figure 3.27(b) and redrawn showing the distance between the individual forces in figure 3.28. By taking moments about the line of action of W_A,

$$\text{CM} = \text{ACM}$$
$$(1.5 \times W_S) + (2.75 \times W_B) = 1.25 \times R$$

Since $W_S = 20 \, \text{kg wt}$ and $W_B = 30 \, \text{kg wt}$ it follows that

$$1.25 \times R = 30 \, \text{m} \cdot \text{kg wt} + 82.5 \, \text{m} \cdot \text{kg wt}$$
$$R = 90 \, \text{kg wt} = W_A + W_S + W_B$$

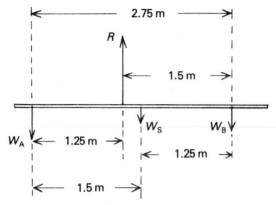

Figure 3.28

Alternatively, by taking moments about the line of action of W_B,

$$CM = ACM$$
$$1.5 \times R = (1.25 \times W_S) + (2.75 \times W_A)$$
$$1.5 \times R = 25\,\text{m.kg wt} + 110\,\text{m.kg wt}$$
$$R = 90\,\text{kg wt}$$

3.4.4 Location of the c. of g. of an object in equilibrium

By equating the clockwise and anticlockwise moments acting on an object which is in equilibrium, the position of the c. of g. of the object (in one plane) can be found. For example, consider Figure 3.29(a) which represents a plank of wood supported in a horizontal position by two knife edges, one of which rests on a set of scales. Figure 3.29(b) shows a free body diagram of the plank of wood. W can be measured by simply weighing the plank of wood. F_A will be equal to the reading on the scales. By taking moments about the knife edge support B,

$$ACM = CM$$
$$W \times D = F_A \times L$$

Therefore,

$$D = \frac{F_A \times L}{W}$$

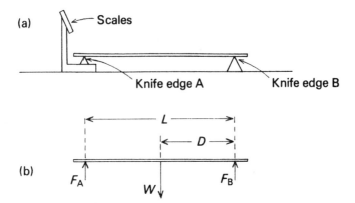

L = Distance between knife edge supports
D = Distance between knife edge B and the position
    of the c. of g. of the plank of wood
W = Weight of the plank of wood
F_A = Force exerted by the knife edge A on the plank
   = Reading on the scales
F_B = Force exerted by knife edge B on the plank

Figure 3.29

For example, if

$$W = 20 \text{ kg wt}$$
$$F_A = 10 \text{ kg wt}$$
$$L = 2.5 \text{ m}$$

then,

$$D = \frac{10 \times 2.5}{20} = 1.25 \text{ m}$$

i.e. the vertical plane containing the c. of g. of the plank of wood lies
a distance of 1.25 m from knife edge B. The apparatus described above
can be used to find the position of the c. of g. of the human body. Figure
3.30(a) shows a man lying down on the plank of wood such that the
soles of his feet and knife edge B lie in the same vertical plane. Figure
3.30(b) shows a free body diagram of the plank of wood. *W*, *L* and *D*

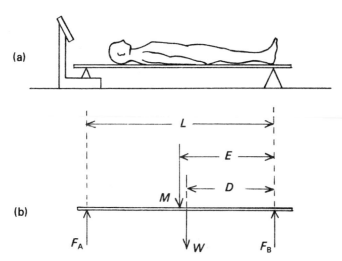

M = Weight of man
E = Distance between vertical plane containing knife edge support B
and the parallel plane containing the c. of g. of the man

Figure 3.30

will be the same as before. However, F_A and F_B will change due to the extra weight of the man acting on the plank of wood. F_A will be equal to the new reading on the scales. By taking moments about knife edge B,

$$ACM = CM$$
$$(W \times D) + (M \times E) = F_A \times L$$
$$E = \frac{(F_A \times L) - (W \times D)}{M}$$

For example, if

$$F_A = 36 \text{ kg wt}$$
$$M = 72 \text{ kg wt}$$
$$W = 20 \text{ kg wt}$$
$$D = 1.25 \text{ m}$$
$$L = 2.5 \text{ m}$$

then,

$$E = \frac{(36 \times 2.5) - (20 \times 2.5)}{72} = 0.904\,\text{m}$$

Therefore, the vertical plane containing the c. of g. of the man lies at a distance of 0.904 m from knife edge B, i.e. 90.4 cm from the soles of his feet.

3.5 The lever
The forces acting on an object are not always parallel forces. For example, consider pulling out a nail from a piece of wood with a claw hammer as shown in Figure 3.31. The nail will be pulled out of the wood

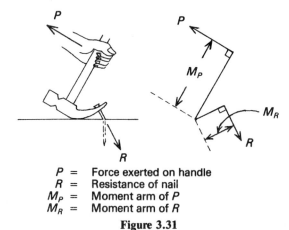

P   =   Force exerted on handle
R   =   Resistance of nail
M_P =   Moment arm of P
M_R =   Moment arm of R

Figure 3.31

if the anticlockwise moment exerted by the man via the handle of the hammer is greater than the clockwise moment exerted by the resistance of the nail. As a further example consider the action of a dinghy sailor in counterbalancing the effect of the wind as shown in Figure 3.32. To prevent the dinghy from capsizing the sailor may need to lean out of the dinghy so that the moment of his weight ($S \times M_S$) in addition to the moment of the weight of the dinghy ($D \times M_D$) can counteract the moment of the wind ($N \times M_N$). Whenever a situation exists in which two forces tend to rotate an object in opposite directions about some specified axis, the object is referred to as a *lever* and the axis as the fulcrum of the lever. One of the forces, usually in the form of a weight or load of some kind, is referred to as the resistance, R. The other force which opposes the turning effect of R is referred to as the effort, E. The simplest form of lever, which is actually the simplest form of

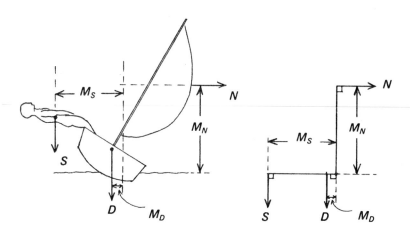

N = Force exerted by wind on sail
D = Weight of dinghy
S = Weight of sailor

M_N = Moment arm of N
M_D = Moment arm of D
M_S = Moment arm of S

Figure 3.32

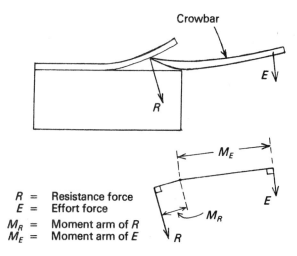

R = Resistance force
E = Effort force

M_R = Moment arm of R
M_E = Moment arm of E

Figure 3.33

machine, is exemplified by the crowbar as shown in Figure 3.33. The greater the moment arm of E (M_E), i.e. the greater the 'leverage', the smaller will be the effort required to overcome the moment of force exerted by the resistance.

Levers are classified into three types according to the positions of the points of application of the effort and resistance forces in relation to the fulcrum. In diagrammatic representations of the different classes of lever it is usual to represent the lever as a straight line, which tends to give the reader the impression that an object acting as a lever must consist of a uniform elongated piece of material such as iron or wood. However, an object acting as a lever can be any shape, as will be demonstrated in the discussion of lever systems within the human body in section 3.5.5. In a diagram of a lever system it is usual to denote the fulcrum as the vertex of a small triangle in contact with the lever, as shown in Figure 3.34(a).

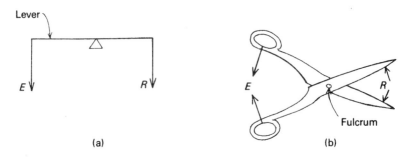

(a)   (b)

Figure 3.34

3.5.1   First-class lever
In a first-class lever system, represented in Figure 3.34(a), the fulcrum is between the E and R forces such as in the crowbar shown in Figure 3.33 and in the seesaw represented in Figure 3.24. A pair of scissors is, in effect, a pair of first-class levers which share the same fulcrum; see Figure 3.34(b).

3.5.2   Second-class lever
In a second-class lever system, represented in Figure 3.35(a), the R force is between the fulcrum and the E force as, for example, in a wheelbarrow; see Figure 3.35(b). A crowbar may also take the form of a second-class lever as shown in Figure 3.35(c).

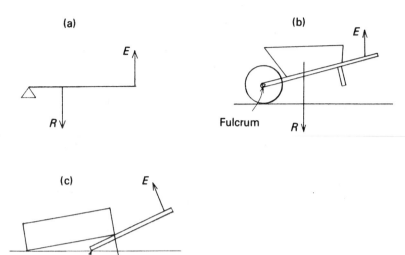

Figure 3.35

3.5.3 Third-class lever

In a third-class lever system, which is represented in Figure 3.36(a), the *E* force is between the fulcrum and the *R* force, as for example when holding a fishing rod; see Figure 3.36(b). A pair of coal tongs is in effect a pair of third-class levers which share the same fulcrum; see Figure 3.36(c).

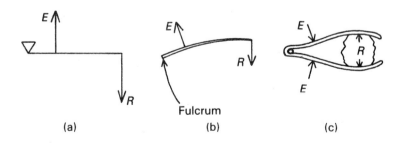

Figure 3.36

3.5.4   Mechanical advantage

The mechanical advantage (MA) of a lever, or any other machine, is a measure of its efficiency in terms of the amount of effort required to move a particular resistance and is given by,

$$MA = \frac{\text{magnitude of resistance}}{\text{magnitude of effort}}$$

$$= \frac{\text{length of effort moment arm } (M_E)}{\text{length of resistance moment arm } (M_R)}$$

Any machine with a MA greater than 1.0 is regarded as very efficient. A first-class lever may have a MA greater or less than 1.0. For example, the MA of the crowbar shown in Figure 3.33 could be made greater or less than 1.0 by varying the length of M_E. Every second-class lever has a MA greater than 1.0 since M_E will always be greater than M_R. In contrast, every third-class lever has a MA less than 1.0 since M_E will always be less than M_R.

3.5.5   Lever systems within the human body

In the human body, the bones of the skeleton act as levers which are rotated about joints by muscles in order to bring about movement. Most, if not all, of the muscles operate within first- or third-class lever systems. There is considerable disagreement as to the existence of any second-class lever systems in the body. Like the third-class levers, most of the first-class lever systems of the body have mechanical advantages less than 1.0 since the tendons of the muscles which operate within them are inserted close to the joints and consequently have short moment arms in relation to the moment arms of the resistance forces they are required to overcome.

An example of a first-class lever system in the body is that of the skull pivoted on top of the vertebral column. The line of action of the weight of the skull passes in front of the vertebral column and in order to maintain the skull in the upright position the extensors of the neck are constantly active; see Figure 3.37.

When the weight of the body is supported by one leg as, for example, during the single leg support phase of walking and running, the pelvis acts as a first-class lever and tends to rotate about the hip joint under the action of body weight and the pull of the hip abductors; see Figure 3.38(a).

Figure 3.38(b) shows a free body diagram of the pelvis, i.e. the forces acting on the pelvis, during a one-legged stance. W will tend to turn the pelvis in a clockwise direction and A will maintain the pelvis in a

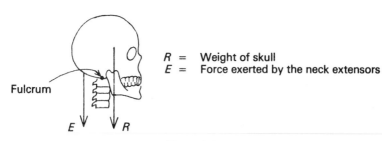

R = Weight of skull
E = Force exerted by the neck extensors

Figure 3.37

horizontal position by exerting an equal and opposite anticlockwise moment. H is the force exerted on the pelvis by the head of the femur. In the body, the line of action of A will be very close to the vertical in a one-legged stance and for demonstration purposes it will be assumed that the line of action of A is vertical. With the pelvis held in a fairly horizontal position as shown in Figure 3.38(b), the clockwise moment exerted by W will be equal and opposite to the anticlockwise moment exerted by A; i.e.,

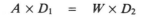

$$A \times D_1 \quad = \quad W \times D_2$$

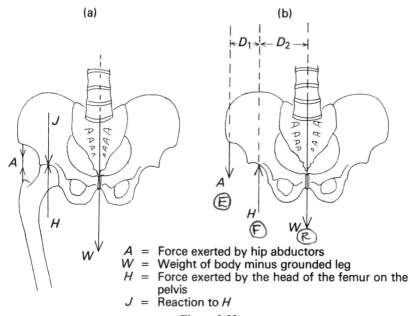

A = Force exerted by hip abductors
W = Weight of body minus grounded leg
H = Force exerted by the head of the femur on the pelvis
J = Reaction to H

Figure 3.38

The force H will have no moment about the hip joint since its line of action passes through the hip joint. D_1 and D_2 will be approximately 7.0 and 11.0 cm, respectively, in the average adult male. For a 70 kg wt man the weight of his body minus the supporting leg will be approximately 59 kg wt (84.4% of total). Therefore, in order to maintain the pelvis in a horizontal position when the weight of the body is supported on one leg, the hip abductors of the supporting leg must exert a force A which is given by,

$$A = \frac{W \times D_2}{D_1} = \frac{59 \times 11}{7} \text{kg wt}$$

$$= 92.7 \text{ kg wt}$$

Since the pelvis is in equilibrium (with respect to the vertical) the resultant of the upward forces acting on the pelvis must be equal and opposite to the resultant of downward forces acting on the pelvis; i.e.,

$$H = A + W$$

$$= 92.7 + 59$$

$$= 151.7 \text{ kg wt}$$

Therefore, the force exerted by the head of the femur on the pelvis is approximately twice body weight when standing on one leg. From Newton's Third Law of Motion, it follows that there will be an equal and opposite force, J, exerted by the pelvis on the head of the femur; see Figure 3.38(a). When a person is learning to walk again during the latter stages of recovering from a fractured femur it is necessary to reduce J as much as possible. As the bone becomes stronger it will be able to take progressively more weight and the use of crutches and later walking sticks will enable the patient to exert more and more weight until the bone is fully recovered. To illustrate the beneficial effect of using a walking stick consider a man walking with the aid of a stick held in his left hand; see Figure 3.39(a).

With his left leg off the ground, the weight of his body will be supported by his right leg and the walking stick. In this example, the left hand, via the left arm and trunk, can be considered to be a lateral extension of the pelvis on the left-hand side such that the forces acting on the very large irregular shaped lever consisting of the whole body minus the supporting leg, which tends to rotate about the right hip joint, can be represented as in Figure 3.39(b). S is the force exerted by the stick on the man's left hand and for the purposes of demonstration it will be assumed that S acts vertically upwards. In the previous

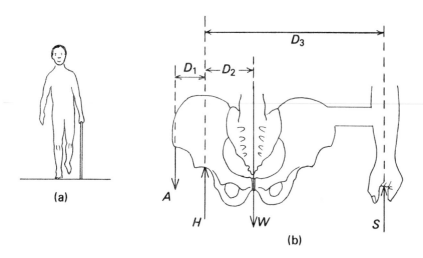

Figure 3.39

example, A acted alone in counterbalancing the moment of W. By using a walking stick, however, the moment of force which counterbalances that of W is made up of two moments, the one provided by A and the one provided by S. By taking moments about the hip joint,

$$A \times D_1 + S \times D_3 \;=\; W \times D_2$$

In the average male, D_3 will be approximately 36.0 cm. S will be approximately 16 kg wt for a man of 70 kg wt. Therefore, the force exerted by the hip abductors when using a walking stick is given by,

$$A \;=\; \frac{W \times D_2 - S \times D_3}{D_1}$$

where $W = 59$ kg wt, $D_1 = 7.0$ cm, $D_2 = 11.0$ cm

$$A \;=\; \frac{(59 \times 11) - (16 \times 36)}{7}$$

$$=\; 10.4 \text{ kg wt}$$

Since the pelvis is in equilibrium (with respect to the vertical) the resultant of the upward forces must be equal and opposite to the downward forces, i.e.

$$H + S = A + W$$
$$H = A + W - S$$
$$= 10.4 + 59 - 16$$
$$= 53.4 \, \text{kg wt}$$

Therefore, the force exerted by the head of the femur on the pelvis is approximately 53.4 kg wt. It follows that the force exerted by the pelvis on the head of the femur is also approximately 53.4 kg wt. These results suggest that by using a walking stick in the contralateral hand, the force exerted by the pelvis on the head of the femur during single leg support is reduced by about two-thirds (from 151.7 to 53.4 kg wt) in comparison with single leg support without the aid of a stick.

The great majority of muscles of the body operate within third-class lever systems. A good example of such a system is the action of the quadriceps on the lower leg in extending the knee joint, as shown in Figure 3.40. Throughout the full range of movement of the joint, the action line of the quadriceps tendon forms an angle of about 20° with the long axis of the lower leg and intersects the long axis of the lower leg approximately 10 cm distal to the axis of the knee joint; see Figure 3.40(b). For a man of stature 170 cm and weight 70 kg wt, the weight of his lower leg and foot will be approximately 4.2 kg wt (6% of total body weight) and the c. of g. of the lower leg and foot will be approximately 20 cm distal to the transverse axis of the knee joint on or near the long axis of the lower leg. With the thigh horizontal and the lower leg held at an angle of 45° to the horizontal as in Figure 3.40(b), the force exerted by the quadriceps can be estimated as follows:

$$M_Q = 10 \sin 20° = 3.42 \, \text{cm}$$
$$M_L = 20 \sin 45° = 14.14 \, \text{cm}$$
$$W_L = 4.2 \, \text{kg wt}$$

Since the thigh and lower leg are in equilibrium,

$$Q \times M_Q = W_L \times M_L$$
$$3.42 \times Q = 59.4$$
$$Q = 17.4 \, \text{kg wt}$$

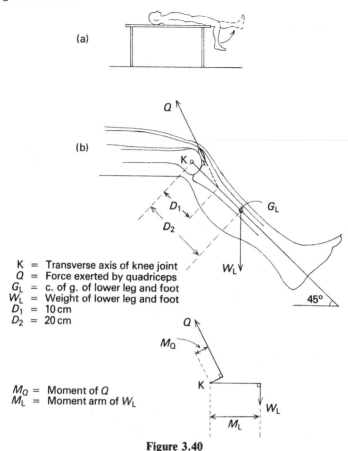

K = Transverse axis of knee joint
Q = Force exerted by quadriceps
G_L = c. of g. of lower leg and foot
W_L = Weight of lower leg and foot
D_1 = 10 cm
D_2 = 20 cm

M_Q = Moment of Q
M_L = Moment arm of W_L

Figure 3.40

Therefore to hold the lower leg and foot at an angle of 45° as shown in Figure 3.40(b), the quadriceps need to exert a force of more than four times the weight of the lower leg and foot. If the knee joint is extended further from the position shown in Figure 3.40(b), M_L will gradually increase, and since W_L does not alter and M_Q is fairly constant throughout the full range of joint movement, the force exerted by the quadriceps will also gradually increase. This force will be maximum when M_L is maximum, i.e. at or near full extension, as shown in Figure 3.41. In this position, the force in the quadriceps is given by,

$$Q = \frac{W_L \times M_L}{M_Q} = \frac{4.2 \times 20}{3.42} = 24.6 \text{ kg wt}$$

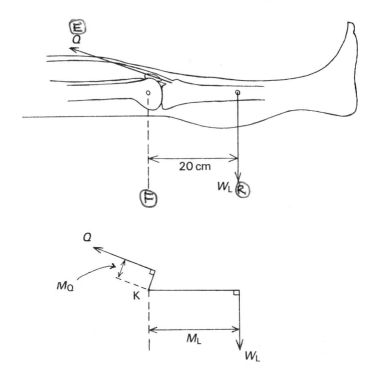

W_L = Weight of lower leg and foot

Figure 3.41

3.6 The application of the principle of moments in selecting training exercises to improve muscle strength and endurance

In any training exercise such as a pull-up, sit-up or press-up the muscles involved are required to overcome a certain amount of resistance in order to perform the exercise. The size of the moment of resistance and, therefore, the training effect on the muscles, can be varied in three ways:

 (i) Altering the moment arm of the weight of the body part which is moved.
 (ii) Increasing the load (resistance force) by adding weights to the body part which is moved.
 (iii) Altering the line of action of the resistance force.

Some examples of the different approaches will now be described.

3.6.1 Trunk curl/sit-up

Consider a man lying on his back with his arms straight and hands, palms down, on the front of his thighs; see Figure 3.42(a). To sit up, his abdominal and hip flexor muscles must overcome the moment of upper body weight about a transverse axis through the hip joints (TAH). The first stage in the sit-up exercise usually involves what is often called a trunk curl, i.e. flexion of the neck and trunk by the neck flexor and abdominal muscles, respectively. This movement results in a decrease in the moment of the upper body weight about the TAH; see Figure 3.42(b). The sit-up is completed by the action of the hip flexors which rotate the upper body about the hips. As the upper body moves from the lying to the sit-up position the moment arm of the upper body weight about the TAH gradually decreases; see Figure 3.42(b) and (c). Therefore, the moment of force necessary to raise the upper body into the sitting position also gradually decreases. Since the moment arm of the hip flexor muscles gradually increases throughout the full range of hip movement, the force exerted by the hip flexors gradually reduces as the upper body assumes the sit-up position. It follows that the most strenuous part of the whole sit-up movement occurs just after the start of hip flexion as the upper body is raised clear of the floor. The sit-up exercise can be made more strenuous by starting with the hands behind the head as shown in Figure 3.42(d). The movement of the arms is in effect a redistribution of the upper body weight such that the moment arm of upper body weight about the TAH is increased (see Figure 3.42(a) and (d); $M_1 < M_2$). Consequently, in raising the upper body into the sitting position, the hip flexors would need to exert a greater force than would be necessary from the previous starting position, as shown in Figure 3.42(a). The exercise could be made even more strenuous by starting with the arms extended above the head as in Figure 3.42(e).

3.6.2 Bent leg sit-up

If the abdominal and hip flexor muscles are not quite strong enough for the individual to perform a sit-up from a starting position with the legs straight (see Figure 3.42(a)), he or she may be able to perform a bent leg sit-up as shown in Figure 3.43. With the hip joints flexed at $45°$ in the starting position as in Figure 3.43(a), the moment arm of the hip flexors is approximately twice as long as when the leg is in the position shown in Figure 3.42(a). Consequently, in raising the upper body into the sitting position, the hip flexors need exert only half as much force when the movement starts from the bent leg position as when starting from the straight leg position. The strain on the abdominal muscles will be about the same whichever starting position is adopted.

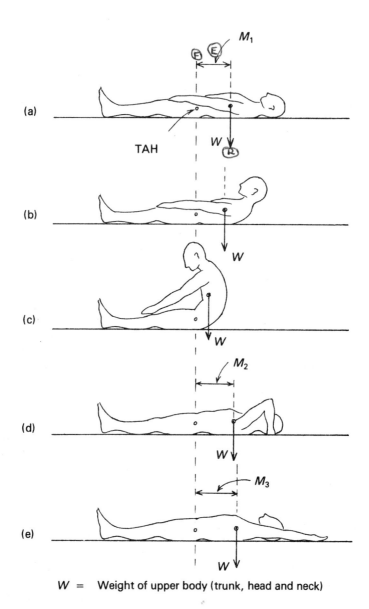

W = Weight of upper body (trunk, head and neck)

Figure 3.42

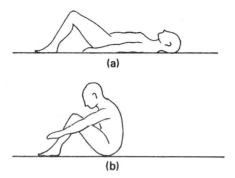

Figure 3.43

3.6.3 Leg Raise

When the hip flexor and, in particular, the abdominal muscles are very weak such that the individual cannot perform even a bent leg sit-up, a suitable exercise to start training these muscles is to raise and lower each leg alternately as shown in Figure 3.44(a) and (b). There is far less strain on both groups of muscles when performing this exercise than when performing a sit-up. The moment arm of the weight of each leg about the TAH is approximately the same as that of the upper body about the TAH after the trunk curl stage of the sit-up movement; see Figures 3.42(b) and 3.44(a). However, since the upper body (minus the arms) and the legs constitute about 56% and 32% respectively of total body weight, the moment of resistance which the hip flexors of each leg need to overcome when performing a single leg-raise is about half of that which must be overcome when performing a sit-up from a starting position with straight legs and about the same as that which must be overcome when performing a sit-up from the bent leg starting position. However, in comparison with this last exercise the strain on the abdominal muscles during a single leg-raise is minimal. The reader might think that a suitable progression from the single leg-raise would be to raise both legs at the same time as shown in Figure 3.44(c). However, in order to perform this exercise correctly, i.e. without the possibility of injury, the abdominal muscles must exert a considerable force in order to prevent the pelvis from tilting forwards (anticlockwise in Figure 3.44). The lower part of the vertebral column forms the rear of the pelvis and if the latter is allowed to tilt forwards, the curve of the lumbar part of the vertebral column is accentuated which may lead to pain and possibly injury if the pelvis is allowed to tilt forwards repetitively during, for example, a number of repetitions of double straight leg-raises.

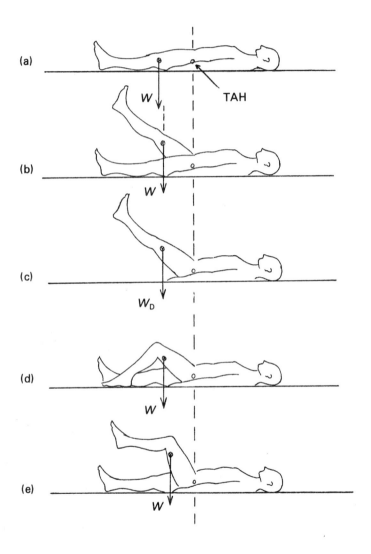

W = Weight of one leg
W_D = Weight of both legs

Figure 3.44

The single leg-raise may be made less strenuous by bending the knee before lifting the leg; see Figure 3.44(d) and (e). Bending the knee has the effect of reducing the moment arm of the leg about the TAH thereby reducing the moment of resistance which the hip flexors must overcome. A suitable progression of exercises for increasing the

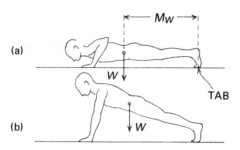

TAB = Transverse axis through balls of feet
W = Body weight
M_W = Moment arm of body weight about TAB

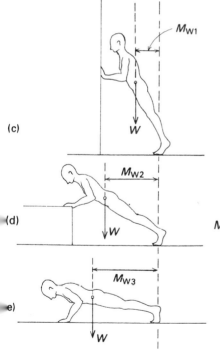

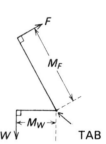

F = Force exerted by the arms
M_F = Moment arm of F about the TAB
$M_{W1} < M_{W2} < M_{W3}$
F increases as M_W increases

Figure 3.45

strength and endurance of the hip flexors and abdominals would be:

- (i) Single bent leg-raise.
- (ii) Double bent leg-raise.
- (iii) Trunk curl.
- (iv) Single straight leg-raise.
- (v) Bent leg sit-up.
- (vi) Straight leg sit-up.
- (vii) Double straight leg-raise.

3.6.4 Press-up (push-up)

During a press-up from the floor, as shown in Figure 3.45(a) and (b), the body segment consisting of head, trunk and legs is held in a straight line and is rotated about the balls of the feet by the action of the arms. To push the body away from the floor the elbow extensors and shoulder flexors must overcome the moment of body weight about the transverse axis through the points of contact between the balls of the feet and the floor (TAB). Consequently the smaller the moment arm of body weight about the TAB the easier the exercise will be in terms of the strain on the elbow extensors and shoulder flexors. Provided the head, trunk and legs are held in the same position relative to each other, the moment arm (M_F) of the force exerted by the arms about the TAB will be more or less the same whatever the inclination of the head, trunk and legs; see Figure 3.45(c–e). However, the greater the inclination of the head, trunk and legs to the vertical, the greater will be the force which the elbow extensors and shoulder flexors must exert in order to extend the arms. Therefore, in order to gradually increase the intensity of the

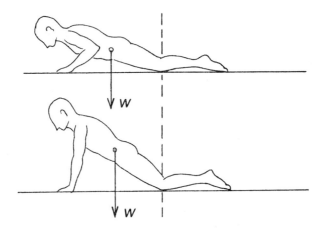

Figure 3.46

press-up exercise the trainee should gradually lower the point of hand support. For example, start with press-ups against a wall (Figure 3.45(c)) and as the strength of the elbow extensors and shoulder flexors increases move on to press-ups against the edge of a table, then a low box or bench (Figure 3.45(d)) and finally against the floor.

Press-ups against the floor can be made less strenuous by using the knees rather than the feet as the fulcrum, as shown in Figure 3.46. In this form of press-up the moment of resistance about the transverse axis through the points of contact between the knees and the floor is considerably less than the moment of resistance about the balls of the feet as in Figure 3.45(a).

3.6.5   Knee extension with a weighted boot

In activities such as running, jumping and throwing the knee extensor muscles – the quadriceps – need to exert very large forces. When an injury to the leg occurs, resulting in a period of inactivity, the muscles of the leg, especially the quadriceps, become much weaker very quickly. In order to strengthen the quadriceps prior to the resumption of fairly strenuous exercise, the trainer may prescribe the knee extension exercise with a weighted boot as shown in Figure 3.47(a). In this form of knee extension exercise, with or without a weighted boot, the moment arm of the resistance force increases as the knee joint extends. Consequently, the most strenuous part of the exercise in terms of the strain on the quadriceps is at full knee extension. Theoretically, there is no strain on the quadriceps when the line of action of the resistance force passes through the knee joint, as shown in position 1 of Figure 3.47(b). In this starting position, with the leg muscles relaxed, the resistance force – the combined weight of lower leg, foot and boot – is supported entirely by the ligaments of the knee joint. These ligaments may be injured if the trainee does not take sufficient care when using a very heavy boot.

It was shown in Section 3.5.5 that for a man of stature 170 cm and weight 70 kg wt, the quadriceps need to exert a force of about 25 kg wt in order to fully extend the knee, as shown in Figure 3.47(c). However, the addition of even a relatively small weight to the lower leg and foot by means of a weighted boot considerably increases the strain and, therefore, the training effect on the quadriceps. The addition of a weighted boot not only increases the resistance force but also increases the moment arm of the resistance force about the transverse axis through the knee joint (TAK); see Figure 3.47(b) and (c). If, for example, the man wears a boot weighing 4.0 kg wt, the resistance force (lower leg, foot and boot) will be approximately 8.0 kg wt. The moment arm of this weight about the TAK will be approximately 35.0 cm. The moment arm of the quadriceps about the TAK will be about 3.5 cm

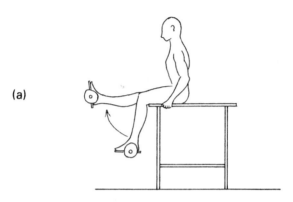

(a)

TAK = Transverse axis through knee joint
  B = Combined weight of lower leg, foot and boot
G_B = Position of c. of g. of B
M_B = Moment arm of B about TAK
  W = Weight of lower leg and foot
G_W = Position of c. of g. of W
M_W = Moment arm of W about TAK

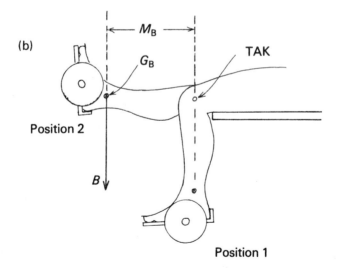

(b)

Figure 3.47

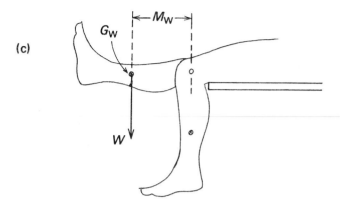

Figure 3.47 *(continued)*

throughout the full range of knee joint movement. Consequently, the force which must be exerted by the quadriceps in order to fully extend the knee, as in Figure 3.47(b), can be estimated as follows:

In full knee extension,

$$Q \times M_Q = B \times M_B$$

where

$$
\begin{array}{rcl}
Q & = & \text{Force exerted by quadriceps} \\
M_Q & = & \text{Moment arm of } Q \text{ about TAK} \\
B & = & \text{Weight of lower leg, foot and boot} \\
M_B & = & \text{Moment arm of } B \text{ about TAK}
\end{array}
$$

$$
\begin{aligned}
Q & = \frac{B \times M_B}{M_Q} \\
& = \frac{8 \times 35}{3.5} \\
& = 80 \, \text{kg wt}
\end{aligned}
$$

In comparison with extending the knee without the addition of extra weight to the lower leg and foot, the addition of a boot weighing 4.0 kg wt increases the strain on the quadriceps by more than three times.

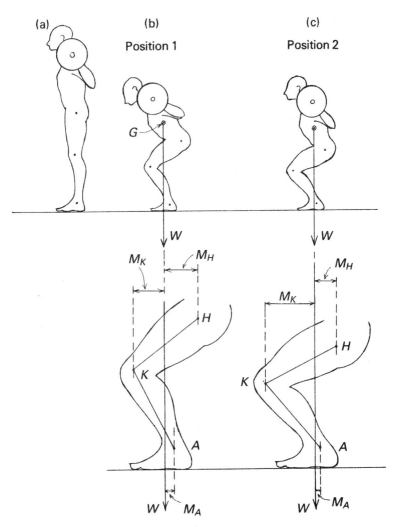

W = Combined weight of barbell and body
G = Position of c. of g. of W
H = Transverse axis through hip joints
K = Transverse axis through knee joints
A = Transverse axis through ankle joints
M_H = Moment arm of W about H
M_K = Moment arm of W about K
M_A = Moment arm of W about A

Figure 3.48

3.6.6 Squat

The squat, as shown in Figure 3.48, is perhaps the most frequently used weight training exercise for increasing the strength and endurance of the leg extensor muscles, i.e. the extensors of the hip, knee and ankle joints. The effect that the exercise has on any one of these three groups of muscles depends upon the moment of resistance about the corresponding joint. Consider, for example, Figure 3.48(b) and (c) which show different body positions for the same depth of squat. With the trunk bent forward as in position 1, the line of action of *W* passes closer to *K* than to *H*. With the trunk held fairly upright as in position 2, the line of action of *W* passes closer to *H* than to *K*. Consequently, the moment of resistance about *H* will be greater in position 1 than in

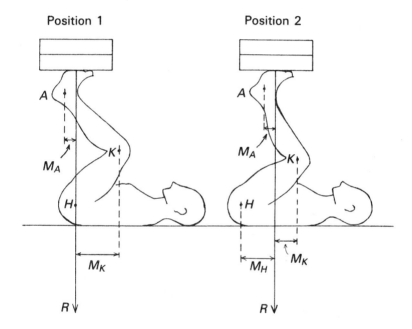

R = Resistance force
A = Transverse axis through the ankle joints
K = Transverse axis through the knee joints
H = Transverse axis through the hip joints
M_A = Moment arm of R about A
M_K = Moment arm of R about K
M_H = Moment arm of R about H

Figure 3.49

position 2. Therefore, the training effect on the hip extensors will be greater in position 1 than in position 2. However, the moment of resistance about *K* will be greater in position 2 than in position 1 and, therefore, the training effect on the knee extensors will be greater in position 2 than in position 1. Since the line of action of *W* passes closer to *A* in position 2 than in position 1, the training effect on the ankle extensors (plantar flexors) will be greater when performing the squat in position 1 than in position 2.

3.6.7 Leg press

In addition to the squat, the leg press is a popular exercise for strengthening the hip, knee and ankle extensors. One form of the leg press requires the trainee to lie on his or her back and push a weight vertically upwards as shown in Figure 3.49. In position 1 the line of action of *R* passes through *H*. Consequently, the main effect of the exercise will be felt by the knee extensors and to a lesser extent the ankle extensors. In position 2, however, the exercise will provide a good training effect for all three muscle groups.

3.7 Angular displacement, angular velocity and angular acceleration

Just as the extent to which an object moves linearly from one place to another is measured by distance travelled, the extent to which an object rotates from one position to another about a particular axis is measured

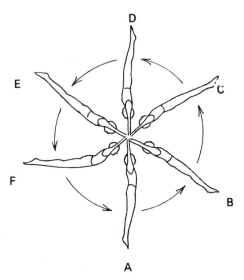

Figure 3.50

by angular distance travelled. Angular distance is usually measured in degrees. There are 360° in one complete revolution. Consider the gymnast in Figure 3.50 performing giant swings on a horizontal bar. By rotating about the bar from position A back to position A he will have travelled an angular distance of 360°. If the direction of rotation is specified, the term angular displacement is used since this incorporates direction of rotation as well as angular distance travelled. In mechanics, angular distance is usually measured in radians rather than in degrees. One radian is defined as the angle subtended at the centre of a circle by an arc which is the same length as the radius of the circle; see Figure 3.51.

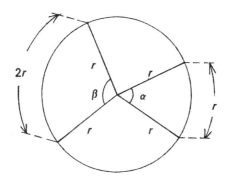

r = Radius of circle
α = 1 radian
β = 2 radians

Figure 3.51

Since $\qquad C = 2\pi r$

where $\qquad C =$ Circumference of circle

$\qquad r =$ Radius of circle

the angular distance travelled
in one revolution $= \dfrac{2\pi r}{r}$ radians

$= 2\pi = 6.2832$ radians

i.e. 1 revolution $= 6.2832$ radians $= 360°$

1 radian $= 57.3°$

The linear speed of an object is defined as the distance travelled by the object per unit of time or the rate of change of distance; i.e.,

$$v = \frac{d}{t}$$

Similarly, the angular speed of a rotating object is defined as the angular distance travelled per unit of time or the rate of change of angular distance; i.e.,

$$\omega = \frac{\theta}{t}$$

where

ω (greek letter omega) = angular speed

θ = angular distance travelled in time t

In mechanics, angular speed is measured in radians per second (rad/s). When the direction of rotation is specified, the term angular velocity is used rather than angular speed.

The linear acceleration of an object is defined as the change in velocity per unit of time or the rate of change of velocity. The angular acceleration of a rotating object is defined as the change in angular velocity per unit of time or the rate of change of angular velocity. For example, if the angular velocity of the gymnast shown in Figure 3.50 increases from 5 rad/s at position E to 15 rad/s at position A in a time of 0.5 s, the average angular acceleration of the gymnast about the bar between positions E and A is given by,

$$\dot{\omega} = \frac{\omega_A - \omega_E}{t}$$

where

$\dot{\omega}$ (pronounced omega dot) = angular acceleration

ω_E = angular velocity at E

= 5 rad/s

ω_A = angular velocity at A

= 15 rad/s

t = 0.5 s

$$\dot{\omega} = \frac{15 - 5}{0.5}$$

$$= 20 \, \text{rad/s}^2$$

3.8 Eccentric force

In the sections on moments and levers, reference was made to objects which were constrained to rotate about a fixed axis or line of contact with some other object. For example, a seesaw can only rotate about an axis through the line of support and a door can only rotate about an axis through its hinges. However, when an object is free to rotate within a particular plane, i.e. not constrained to rotate about any fixed axis or line contact with another object, and a force acts on the object which causes the object to rotate, the rotation will take place about an axis which passes through the c. of g. of the object. To illustrate this principle, consider a man pushing a vaulting box across a gymnasium floor. Assuming the box does not tip over onto its side, the movement of the box will be confined within a horizontal plane – the plane of the floor. If the line of action of the man's push is directed through the c. of g. of the box, the box will not rotate but move in the direction of the push as shown in Figure 3.52(a); the box will be translated.

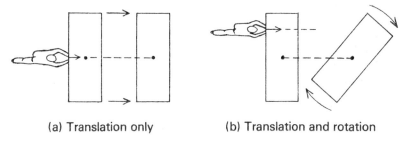

(a) Translation only   (b) Translation and rotation

Figure 3.52

However, if the line of action of the push is 'off centre' or 'eccentric', i.e. if it does not pass through the c. of g. of the box, a turning moment will be created about the vertical axis passing through the c. of g. of the box, such that the box will rotate about this axis. Simultaneously, the c. of g. of the box will move in a straight line parallel to the line of action of the push; see Figure 3.52(b). Therefore, the box will be simultaneously translated and rotated. Any force which causes or tends to cause simultaneous translation and rotation of an object is called an *eccentric force*.

In many gymnastic and athletic movements which involve rotation of the body, the direction of the ground reaction at take-off will be eccentric to the performer's c. of g. For example, consider Figure 3.53

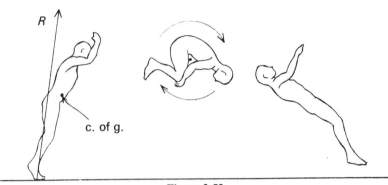

Figure 3.53

which shows a gymnast performing a front somersault following a run-up. Just prior to take-off, the line of action of the ground reaction passes behind the gymnast's c. of g. The effect of the ground reaction force will be to simultaneously lift the gymnast's c. of g. (i.e. move the c. of g. in a straight line parallel to the line of action of the ground reaction) and help create forward rotation of his or her body during the flight phase about a transverse axis through the gymnast's c. of g.

Similarly, in the final stages of a headspring, the line of action of the thrust resulting from arm, wrist and finger extension passes behind the c. of g. of the body; see Figure 3.54. The turning moment thus created helps to increase forward rotation of the body during the flight phase about a transverse axis through the body's c. of g. and consequently increases the chances of the performer landing on the feet.

Another example of the effect of an eccentric force can often be seen in the flight of a rugby ball. If the ball is kicked such that the line of action of the kick passes through the c. of g. of the ball, then the ball

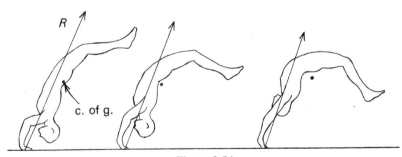

Figure 3.54

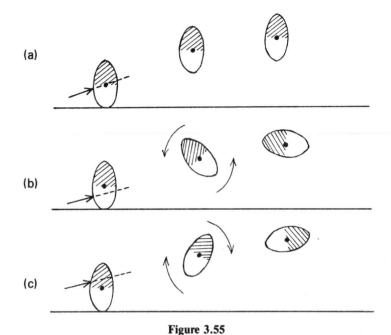

Figure 3.55

will travel through the air without any rotation; see Figure 3.55(a). However, if the line of action of the kick passes below the c. of g. of the ball, the ball will rotate backwards about a transverse axis through its c. of g. as it travels through the air; see Figure 3.55(b). If the line of action of the kick passes above the c. of g. of the ball, which is often referred to as 'topping' the ball, the ball will rotate forwards as it travels through the air; see Figure 3.55(c).

3.9   Couple

Figure 3.56(a) shows two gymnasts trying to turn a vaulting box through some particular angle. Each gymnast applies an eccentric force to the box tending to rotate it in the same direction, clockwise in Figure 3.56(a).

If the forces exerted by the gymnasts are equal and parallel the translatory effects of both forces will cancel each other out such that the box will rotate about a vertical axis through its c. of g. which will remain over the same spot on the floor; see Figure 3.56(b). Any system of two parallel, equal and opposite eccentric forces acting on an object is called a *couple*. The magnitude of a couple is the product of one of

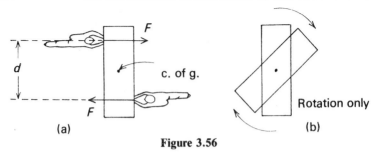

Figure 3.56

the forces and the perpendicular distance between the forces; in Figure 3.56(a), the magnitude of the couple C acting on the box is given by,

$$C = Fd$$

The larger the couple acting on an object, the greater will be the angular acceleration and, therefore, the speed of rotation of the object.

As a further illustration, consider the movement of a child's roundabout as shown from above in Figure 3.57. If the roundabout did not rest on a vertical support but was free to rotate within a horizontal plane, the effect of an eccentric force, F, applied by a child to the roundabout via one of the handrails would be a tendency for the roundabout to rotate about a vertical axis through its c. of g. and for the

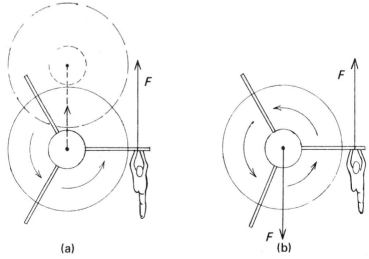

Figure 3.57

c. of g. to move in in a straight line parallel to the line of action of F; see Figure 3.57(a). However, since a roundabout normally rests on a vertical support so that it can only rotate about a vertical axis through its point of support, the tendency of F to move the c. of g. of the round-about in the direction of F would be counteracted by an equal and opposite force F exerted by the point of support on the roundabout; see Figure 3.57(b). The force F exerted by the child and the counter-acting force F exerted by the vertical support on the roundabout con-stitute a couple, such that the roundabout rotates about a fixed vertical axis through the point of support.

The concepts expressed in Sections 3.8 and 3.9 regarding the con-ditions in which an object is translated, rotated or simultaneously translated and rotated may be summarised as follows:

(i) Consider an object which is free to rotate within a particular plane, i.e. not constrained to rotate about any particular axis or line of contact with another object.

(a) If the object is acted upon by a force, parallel to the plane of movement, whose line of action passes through the axis A_G which is perpendicular to the plane of movement and which passes through the c. of g. of the object, the object will be translated in the plane of movement but will not rotate.

(b) If the object is acted upon by a force, parallel to the plane of movement, whose line of action does not pass through the axis A_G, the object will be simultaneously translated and rotated, i.e. the object will rotate about A_G and A_G will move (translate) in space. Such a force is called an eccentric force.

The effect of an eccentric force, F, acting at a distance, d, from the axis A_G (as defined above) is the same as the combined effect of a couple of magnitude Fd and a force F, parallel to the eccentric force, whose line of action passes through A_G. For example, consider a man pushing a box across a gymnasium floor as shown in Figure 3.58. The only force acting on the box in a horizontal plane is the force F_1

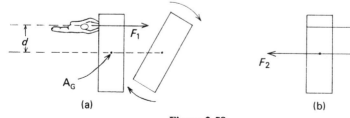

(a) (b)

Figure 3.58

exerted by the man; see Figure 3.58(a). If F_1 is eccentric to the vertical axis A_G passing through the c. of g. of the box and the box is free to rotate within the horizontal plane, the box will simultaneously rotate about A_G and translate as shown in Figure 3.58(a). The effect of the single force $F1$ can be more easily appreciated, perhaps, if it is thought to set up two equal and opposite forces F_2 and F_3, both of equal magnitude to F_1, acting at the c. of g. of the box and parallel to F_1; see Figure 3.58(b). This new three-force system has the same effect as the single force F_1 since F_2 and F_3 cancel each other out. However, it can be seen that F_1 and F_2 set up a couple of magnitude F_1d which causes the box to rotate about A_G clockwise in Figure 3.58. Simultaneously, F_3 translates the box.

(ii) When the forces acting on an object cause it to rotate about an axis which does not move (translate) in space, the resultant of the forces responsible for the rotation will be in the form of a couple – two parallel, equal and opposite eccentric forces.

3.10   Rotation and Newton's First Law of Motion

It will be evident from the previous section that a non-rotating object will begin to rotate about a particular axis only when the resultant force acting on the object is an eccentric force or a couple. Newton's laws of motion apply to angular motion as well as linear motion and at this stage it will be worthwhile to make an analogy between the effect of Newton's first law on the two forms of motion. With regard to linear motion, the law may be expressed as follows:

> *Every object will remain at rest or continue with uniform*
> *linear velocity unless acted upon by an unbalanced force.*

With regard to angular motion, the law may be expressed in a similar way:

> *Every object will remain in a non-rotating state, or will*
> *continue to rotate about a particular axis with uniform*
> *angular velocity,* unless acted upon by an unbalanced*
> *eccentric force or couple.*

To illustrate the effect of this law on angular motion, consider a bicycle turned upside down so that it rests on the saddle and handlebars; see Figure 3.59(a). Each wheel will remain in a state of non-rotation unless an eccentric force or couple (with respect to the wheel spindle) is applied to it. When the pedals are turned anticlockwise with respect to Figure 3.59(a), the chain will transmit an eccentric force to the back wheel such

---

* Provided that the shape of the object stays the same; see Sections 3.11 and 3.12.

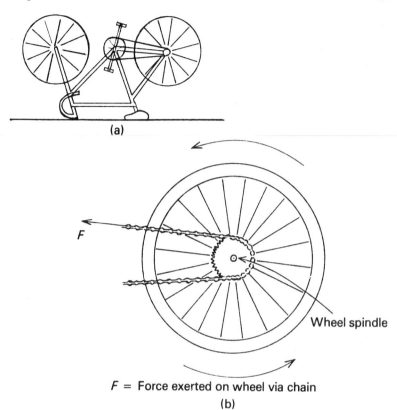

F = Force exerted on wheel via chain

(b)

Figure 3.59

that the wheel will start to rotate; see Figure 3.59(b). When the pedals are brought to rest, the wheel will continue to rotate (provided that it is not a 'fixed wheel'). Furthermore, the wheel will continue to rotate for some time unless a counter-rotation eccentric force, in the form of a brake, is applied to the wheel. If a brake is not applied to the wheel, the amount of time that it will continue to rotate will depend upon the amount of friction between the wheel and the spindle. If this source of friction could be reduced to zero, the wheel would continue to rotate *for ever with uniform angular velocity*, provided no braking force was applied to it. In effect, the friction between wheel and spindle exerts a counter-rotation eccentric force on the wheel; the greater the friction, the sooner the wheel will be brought to rest.

In movements such as somersaults, in which the human body rotates freely in space during the flight phase of the movement, the rotation of the body will take place about the axis which passes through the c. of g. of the body. Furthermore, the angular velocity of the body about its axis of rotation will be constant provided that the orientation of the different parts of the body to each other does not alter. The rotation of the body in such movements is ultimately destroyed by the action of the ground reaction (an unbalanced eccentric force) on landing.

3.11 Moment of inertia

The reluctance of a resting object to start moving linearly is referred to as its inertia. The inertia of an object is directly proportional to its mass; the larger the mass, the greater the inertia. The reluctance or resistance of an object to start rotating about a particular axis is referred to as its *moment of inertia*. The moment of inertia of an object about a particular axis depends not only on the mass of the object but also on the distribution of the mass of the object about the axis of rotation. The closer the mass of the object to the axis of rotation or the more concentrated the mass of the object about the axis of rotation, the smaller will be the moment of inertia of the object and the easier it will be to start the object rotating, i.e. the smaller the turning moment which will be required to start the object rotating. Consider Figure 3.60 which shows two positions of a gymnast performing a forward giant circle on a horizontal bar. The human body or any other object can be considered to consist of any number of separate masses joined together. Consider the motion of a tiny particle *m* of the gymnast's

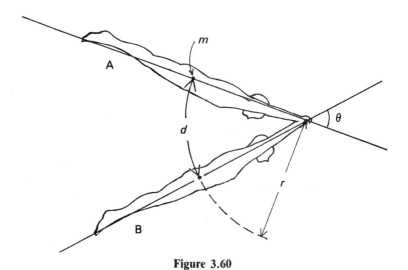

Figure 3.60

mass. If the orientation of the gymnast's body parts to each other remains the same in moving from position A to position B, the average linear velocity v of the particle during this period is given by,

$$v = \frac{d}{t} \tag{1}$$

where

d = Distance travelled by m

t = Time taken to travel from position A to position B

The average angular velocity of the particle about the axis of rotation during the same period is given by,

$$\omega = \frac{\theta}{t} \tag{2}$$

where

θ = Angular distance travelled by m with respect to the axis of rotation

Since θ degrees = d/r radians, where r is the radius of the circle along which m travels,

$$d = r\theta \tag{3}$$

By substitution of (3) into (1),

$$v = \frac{r\theta}{t} = r\omega$$

i.e., the average linear velocity of the particle in moving from position A to position B is equal to the product of the distance of the particle from the axis of rotation and the average angular velocity of the particle during the same period. Therefore,

$$v_A = r\omega_A \quad \text{and} \quad v_B = r\omega_B$$

where v_A, v_B and ω_A, ω_B are the linear and angular velocities of the particle at positions A and B. The linear acceleration a of the particle in moving from position A to position B is given by,

$$a = \frac{v_B - v_A}{t} = \frac{r(\omega_B - \omega_A)}{t}$$

Since $(\omega_B - \omega_A)/t = \dot{\omega}$ = angular acceleration of the particle in moving from position A to position B,

$$a \ = \ r\dot{\omega}$$

From Newton's Second Law of Motion, the force F responsible for the linear acceleration of the particle is given by,

$$F \ = \ ma$$

Since $a = r\dot{\omega}$,

$$F \ = \ mr\dot{\omega} \tag{4}$$

The turning moment of the force F about the axis of rotation is equal to Fr, i.e.,

$$Fr \ = \ mr^2\dot{\omega} \tag{5}$$

The total or resultant turning moment of all the forces acting on the body is given by,

$$\text{Resultant moment} \ = \ F_1 r_1 + F_2 r_2 + F_3 r_3 + \ldots F_n r_n$$

where n is the number of particles which make up the whole body. Since the axis of rotation is fixed, i.e. the position of the bar does not alter, the resultant moment is a couple C such that,

$$\begin{aligned} C \ &= \ F_1 r_1 + F_2 r_2 + \ldots F_n r_n \\ &= \ m_1 r_1^2 \dot{\omega} + m_2 m_2^2 \dot{\omega} + \ldots m_n r_n^2 \dot{\omega} \\ &= \ \left(\sum_{n=1}^{n=n} m_n r_n^2 \right) \dot{\omega} \end{aligned}$$

The term $\left(\sum_{n=1}^{n=n} m_n r_n^2 \right)$ is called the moment of inertia of the body about the axis of rotation and is usually denoted by the capital letter I; i.e.,

$$C \ = \ I\dot{\omega}$$

The moment of inertia of a body about any axis is thus obtained by multiplying the mass of each particle of the body by the square of its perpendicular distance from the axis of rotation and adding them up

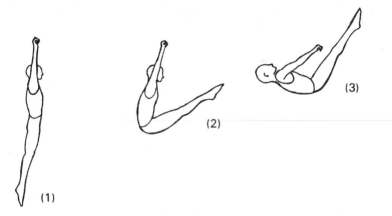

Figure 3.61

for the whole body. As the distribution of the mass of an object about a particular axis alters, so will the distance of each particle of mass of the object from the axis of rotation. Consequently, the moment of inertia of the object about the axis of rotation will also change. Consider Figure 3.61 which shows three possible positions of a gymnast rotating about a horizontal bar. In position 1 the mass of the gymnast is distributed as far away as possible from the axis of rotation. Consequently, the moment of inertia of the body about this particular axis of rotation will be maximum in position 1. In position 2, the legs are much closer to the bar than in position 1 such that the moment of inertia of the body about the bar will be smaller in position 2 than in position 1. In position 3, the trunk and legs are much closer to the bar than in positions 1 and 2 such that the moment of inertia of the body about the bar will be smaller in position 3 than in positions 1 and 2. In the metric system, moment of inertia is measured in kilogram–metre squared units ($kg.m^2$). The moment of inertia of an object rotating about a particular axis is the same as that of a very thin ring of material of radius K and of mass M equal to that of the object, which rotates about an axis which is perpendicular to the plane of the ring and which passes through the centre of the ring; see Figure 3.62. Hence:

$$I = \sum_{n=1}^{n=n} m_n r_n^2 = MK^2$$

The length K is called the radius of gyration of the object about the axis of rotation. The moment of inertia of an object about a particular axis

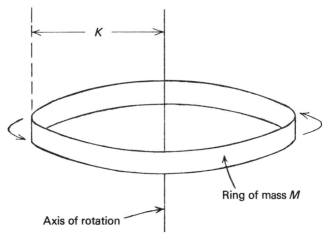

Figure 3.62

is usually expressed in terms of MK^2. For a given object, M is constant but the length K and, therefore, the moment of inertia of the object depend upon the distribution of the mass of the object about the axis of rotation.

3.12   Angular momentum
Just as an object moving with linear velocity has a certain linear momentum, a rotating object has a certain *angular momentum* about its axis of rotation. The angular momentum of an object about a particular axis of rotation is the product of its moment of inertia and angular velocity about the axis of rotation; i.e.,

$$\text{Angular momentum} \quad = \quad I\omega$$
$$\text{Linear momentum} \quad = \quad mv$$

where m = mass and v = linear velocity. Whereas the mass of an object cannot change (other than by chopping off some of the mass of the object), the moment of inertia of a rotating object can be changed simply by redistributing the mass of the object about the axis of rotation. From Newton's First Law of Motion, the angular momentum of an object about a particular axis will remain constant unless the object is acted upon by an unbalanced eccentric force or couple. Therefore, if the moment of inertia of an object rotating freely about a particular axis is altered, there will be a simultaneous change in the

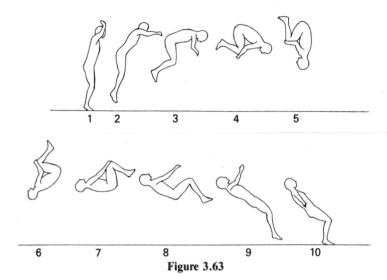

Figure 3.63

angular velocity of the object so that the angular momentum of the object remains the same as before. This principle is referred to as the *conservation of angular momentum* and it has great significance in a number of gymnastic and athletic activities. For example, consider Figure 3.63 which shows the successive positions of a gymnast during the performance of a front somersault following a run-up. The drawings are taken from film and the time between successive positions is 1/32 s. During the flight period – positions 2–9 – the gymnast rotates in the median plane about a transverse axis through his or her c. of g. (TAG). Since there are no unbalanced turning forces acting on the gymnast whilst in flight, the angular momentum of the gymnast about the TAG will remain constant.

To land on the feet, the gymnast must complete the forward somersault very quickly, i.e. he must rotate about the TAG very quickly. By tucking the body (positions 2–4) the gymnast reduces the moment of inertia about the TAG which simultaneously results in an increase in angular velocity about the TAG. Suppose that in position 5 the moment of inertia of the gymnast about the TAG is only half of that in position 2. Since the angular momentum of the gymnast about the TAG is the same in positions 2 and 5,

$$I_2\omega_2 \ = \ I_5\omega_5$$

where I_2, I_5 and ω_2, ω_5 are the moments of inertia and angular velocities of the gymnast in positions 2 and 5.

If $I_5 = I_2/2$ then

$$I_2\omega_2 = \frac{I_2}{2}\omega_5$$

Therefore,

$$\omega_5 = 2\omega_2$$

i.e. by halving the moment of inertia about the TAG, the gymnast has doubled the angular velocity. The increased angular velocity will enable the gymnast to complete the forward somersault quickly and thereby allow more time to prepare a good landing. In the last part of the movement (positions 7–9) the gymnast opens out the body, increasing the moment of inertia about the TAG and simultaneously decreasing the angular velocity in preparation for landing. Figure 3.64 shows the relationship between I and ω about the TAG during the flight phase of the movement.

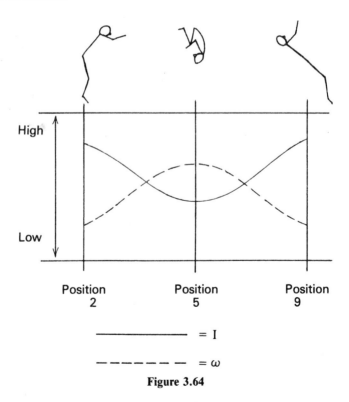

Figure 3.64

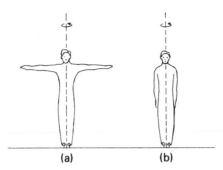

Figure 3.65

Another example of the effect of the conservation of angular momentum is afforded by a skater rotating about a vertical axis as shown in Figure 3.65. If the skater goes into a spin with the arms outstretched at the sides, as in Figure 3.65(a), and then suddenly brings in the arms close to the sides, as in Figure 3.65(b), the moment of inertia of the skater's body about the vertical axis of rotation will be reduced and consequently angular velocity about the axis will increase. In this movement, angular momentum about the vertical axis is not entirely conserved since the friction between the skates and ice will exert a small counter-rotation turning moment such that if the skater could continue to spin about the vertical axis, angular momentum would gradually be reduced to zero; the skater would eventually stop spinning. The reader can experience the changes in angular velocity resulting from changes in the moment of inertia of the body about a vertical axis by using a chair, stool or turntable which is free to rotate about a vertical axis. With subject and chair rotating as in Figure 3.66(a), movement of the arms and/or the legs away from the vertical axis of rotation

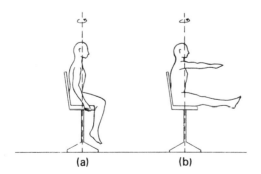

Figure 3.66

will result in a decrease in angular velocity and vice versa. The effect is more marked if the subject holds weights in the hands or wears weighted shoes since movement of 'heavier' limbs results in more marked changes in the moment of inertia of the body about the axis of rotation. The angular momentum of subject and chair is not entirely conserved since there will be a certain amount of friction between the chair and its spindle.

3.13 Rotation and Newton's Second Law of Motion

It was shown in Section 3.11 that when an unbalanced turning moment, in the form of a couple or the 'couple component' of an eccentric force acts on an object, the angular acceleration experienced by the object about an axis perpendicular to the plane of the turning moment is directly proportional to the magnitude of the turning moment and inversely proportional to the moment of inertia of the object about the axis of rotation; i.e.,

$$\dot{\omega} \;=\; \frac{Fd}{I} \tag{1}$$

where

$$Fd \;=\; \text{turning moment}$$

This equation represents Newton's Second Law of Motion as it relates to rotation. The law may be expressed as follows:

> *When an unbalanced turning moment results in rotating an object about a particular axis, the angular acceleration experienced by the object takes place in the direction of the turning moment and is proportional to the magnitude of the turning moment and inversely proportional to the moment of inertia of the object about the axis of rotation.*

It should be realised that the direction of an unbalanced turning moment acting on a rotating object will determine whether the angular velocity of the object is increased or decreased. If the turning moment acts in the same direction as that of the rotating object, then the angular velocity of the object will be increased. However, if the turning moment acts in the opposite direction to that of the rotating object, the turning moment will act as a brake and the angular velocity of the object will be decreased. The amount of change in angular momentum depends not only on the direction of the turning moment in relation to that of the rotating object but also on the length of time that the turning moment is applied.

From equation (1),

$$Fd = I\dot{\omega}$$

Since

$$\dot{\omega} = (\omega_2 - \omega_1)/t$$

where

t = the length of time that the turning moment is applied

and

ω_1, ω_2 = the angular velocities of the object at the start and end of the application of the turning moment

it follows that,

$$Fd = I(\omega_2 - \omega_1)/t$$

$$\text{i.e.} \quad Fdt = I(\omega_2 - \omega_1) \tag{2}$$

Newton's second law is often expressed in terms of equation (2), as follows:

> *When an unbalanced turning moment results in rotating an object about a particular axis, the change in angular momentum experienced by the object takes place in the direction of the turning moment and is directly proportional to the magnitude of the turning moment and the length of time that the turning moment is applied.*

Hence to give an object maximum angular velocity about a particular axis it is necessary to apply as much turning moment as possible for as long as possible. When a turning moment acts on an object the product of the turning moment and the length of time that the turning moment is applied is called the impulse of the turning moment. The impulse principle is used to good effect in a number of gymnastic movements, especially those which involve rotation of the body about a transverse axis through the c. of g. of the body. For example, consider Figure 3.67 which shows four successive body positions of a gymnast immediately prior to take-off during the performance of a standing back somersault. During the pre-take-off period the gymnast needs to generate vertical thrust in order to lift the gymnast off the floor and backward rotation about the transverse axis through his or her c. of g. These requirements are met by a ground reaction force which passes in front of the c. of g. of the body. The greater the speed of leg extension, the greater the ground reaction force and consequently the greater the

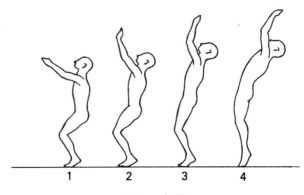

Figure 3.67

turning moment. In order to maximise the length of time that the turning moment operates, it is necessary to maintain contact with the floor for as long as possible. This is achieved by fully extending the hip, knee and ankle joints and flexing the toe joints prior to take-off. Figure 3.68 shows four successive body positions of a gymnast immediately

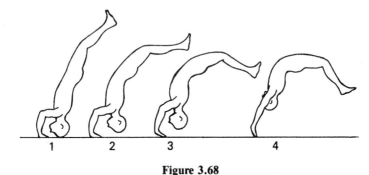

Figure 3.68

prior to take-off during the performance of a headspring. In order to land on his or her feet the gymnast needs to generate forward angular momentum about a transverse axis through the c. of g. This is achieved by a ground reaction force which passes in front of his or her c. of g. The impulse of the turning moment thus created is maximised by rapid and full extension of the elbow joints and rapid and full flexion of the shoulders, wrists and fingers.

3.14 Transfer of angular momentum

From Newton's Second Law of Motion, the acceleration $\dot{\omega}$ experienced by an object subjected to a turning moment Fd is given by,

$$\dot{\omega} = \frac{Fd}{I}$$

where I = Moment of inertia of the object about the axis of rotation. As shown in Section 3.11,

$$I\dot{\omega} = (m_1r_1^2)\dot{\omega} + (m_2r_2^2)\dot{\omega} + \ldots (m_nr_n^2)\dot{\omega}$$

where $m_1 m_2, \ldots m_n$ are the particles of mass which constitute the whole mass of the object, and $r_1, r_2, \ldots r_n$ are the respective distances of the particles of mass from the axis of rotation. Since $\dot{\omega} = \omega/t$, where ω = angular velocity of object after time t,

$$\frac{I\omega}{t} = (m_1r_1^2)\frac{\omega}{t} + (m_2r_2^2)\frac{\omega}{t} + \ldots (m_nr_n^2)\frac{\omega}{t}$$

$$I\omega = (m_1r_1^2)\omega + (m_2r_2^2)\omega + \ldots (m_nr_n^2)\omega$$

$$= I_1\omega + I_2\omega + \ldots I_n\omega$$

where $I_1, I_2, \ldots I_n$ are the respective moments of inertia of the particles about the axis of rotation. It follows, therefore, that the angular momentum of the object about the axis of rotation is equal to the sum of the angular momenta of all the individual particles of mass which constitute the whole mass of the object. Consequently, when an object is rotating with constant angular momentum about a particular axis, any change (increase, decrease) in the angular momentum of one or more parts of the object as a result of internal forces will simultaneously result in a change (decrease, increase) in the angular momentum of the rest of the object so that the angular momentum of the object remains unchanged. For example, consider Figure 3.69(a) which shows a man standing with his arms outstretched at his sides on a turntable which is free to rotate about a vertical axis V_S.

If the turntable is rotated by an external turning moment which is then removed, the system (composite body) consisting of man and turntable will continue to rotate with constant angular momentum about the vertical axis V_S; see Figure 3.69(b–d). If the man suddenly moves his left arm relative to the rest of the system, in a horizontal plane, and in the direction of the whole system, the angular velocity of the rest of the system about V_S will be seen to be reduced for the same period of

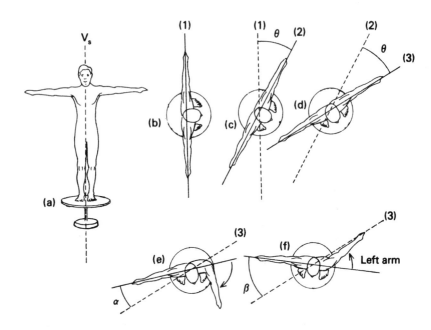

Figure 3.69   The time period between the positions shown in (b) and (c), (c) and (d), (d) and (e), and (d) and (f) is the same

time that the left arm is moving relative to the rest of the system. In the same time that it takes the left arm to move through 90° about a vertical axis through the shoulder joint, the rest of the system moves through a smaller angle about V_S than it would have done if the left arm had not moved relative to the rest of the body; see Figure 3.69(d) and (e), where $\alpha < \theta$. The angular momentum of the whole system about V_S is equal to the sum of the angular momentum of the left arm about V_S and the angular momentum of the rest of the system about V_S. Since the movement of the left arm relative to the rest of the body results in a decrease in the angular momentum of the rest of the system about V_S, it follows that there must be a simultaneous increase in the angular momentum of the left arm about V_S so that the angular momentum of the whole system about V_S is conserved. In effect, the movement of the left arm *relative to the rest of the body* results in a transfer of angular momentum from the rest of the body to the left arm, *for as long as the left arm is moving relative to the rest of the body.* If the left arm is moved, relative to the rest of the body, in the direction of rotation of the whole system, then angular momentum will be transferred from the rest of the system to the left arm. However, if the left arm is moved in the opposite direction to that of the whole system, angular momentum will be transferred from the left arm to the rest of the system; the angular velocity of the rest of the system about V_S will be seen to increase during the same period that the left arm is moving relative to the rest of the body; see Figure 3.69(d) and (f), where $\beta > \theta$.

It is evident that for an object such as the human body which consists of a number of joined segments which are able to move relative to each other, angular momentum can be transferred from one segment of the object to another by the action of internal forces exerted between the joined segments. The angular momentum of any particular segment can be increased/decreased by increasing/decreasing the angular velocity of the segment relative to the axis of rotation of the whole system. *The principle of transfer of angular momentum* can be most clearly demonstrated, perhaps, by using a turntable which is free to rotate about a vertical axis V_S and a bicycle wheel which has handles attached to the ends of its spindle so that the wheel can rotate independently of the handles. A man stands on the turntable and holds the wheel, with its spindle vertical, in one hand as shown in Figure 3.70. If the turntable is then rotated by an external turning moment which is subsequently removed, the whole system (man, turntable and wheel) will continue to rotate about V_S with constant angular momentum. If the man then rotates the wheel about its spindle in the direction of

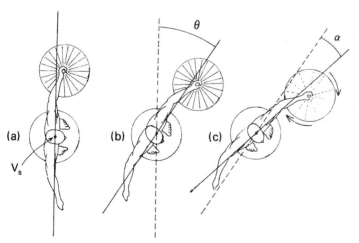

Figure 3.70 The time period between the positions shown in (a) and (b) and (b) and (c) is the same

rotation of the whole system, the angular velocity and, therefore, the angular momentum of the rest of the system, i.e. man and turntable about V_S will decrease; see Figure 3.70(b) and (c), where $\alpha < \theta$. Since the angular momentum of the whole system about V_S is conserved, the angular momentum lost by the man and turntable is gained by the wheel; by rotating the wheel in the direction of rotation of the whole system, angular momentum is transferred from the man and turntable to the wheel. If the man then stops the wheel rotating by touching it against his chest, the whole system will start to rotate about V_S with the same angular velocity as at the start of the experiment, i.e. after the removal of the external turning moment. Therefore, by stopping the wheel from rotating, angular momentum is transferred back from the wheel to the rest of the system. The principle of transfer of angular momentum is of great significance in many gymnastic and athletic movements. For example, consider Figure 3.71 which shows four successive positions of a diver performing a forward piked dive. The diver leaves the board with a certain amount of forward angular momentum about the transverse axis through his c. of g. (TAG). The angular momentum is the result of the ground reaction force passing behind the diver's c. of g. prior to take-off. Just after take-off, the diver bends

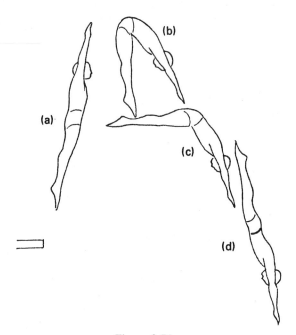

Figure 3.71

forward his upper body (trunk, head and arms) and achieves the piked position as shown in Figure 3.71(b). The act of bending the upper body forward (flexing hip joints) increases the angular velocity of the upper body relative to the TAG which increases the angular momentum of this segment about the TAG. Since the angular momentum of the whole body about the TAG is conserved during the flight phase, an increase in the angular momentum of the upper body must result in a decrease in the angular momentum of the rest of the body, i.e. the legs. This is in fact what happens in the piked dive. The increase in angular momentum of the upper body is gained at the expense of the legs, the angular velocity relative to the TAG and angular momentum about the TAG of which are decreased. If the piking action is carried out very rapidly, i.e. if angular velocity of the upper body relative to the TAG is considerably increased, the angular velocity of the legs relative to the TAG may be reduced to zero or the direction of rotation of the legs may even be reversed as shown in Figure 3.71(b) (compare with Figure 3.71(a)). In the latter stages of the piked dive, the diver needs to straighten out his body in preparation for entry into the water; see Figure 3.71(c) and (d). As the body straightens out (due to hip extension) the angular velocity of the legs relative to the TAG is increased which results in an increase in the angular momentum of the legs about the TAG. Since the angular momentum of the whole body about the TAG is conserved the gain in angular momentum of the legs about the TAG is at the expense of the upper body whose angular velocity relative to the TAG is decreased. In the time it takes the body position to change from that shown in Figure 3.71(b) to that shown in Figure 3.71(d) the legs rotate through about 180° while the upper body rotates through a much smaller angle of about 25°.

The hitch-kick technique of long jumping is a good example of the application of the principle of transfer of angular momentum in order to improve performance. At take-off the jumper wants maximum horizontal velocity and maximum vertical velocity. Horizontal velocity is achieved largely by the run-up, but vertical velocity can be achieved only by pushing down hard on the take-off board with the trailing leg. As a result of the downward push, the ground reaction tends to pass behind the jumper's c. of g.; see Figure 3.72(a). The near vertical eccentric ground reaction force generates not only upward velocity of the jumper's c. of g. but also forward angular momentum of the jumper's body about the transverse axis through the c. of g. (TAG); the angular momentum will be conserved during the flight phase of the jump. If the jumper does not alter the orientation of his or her body parts to each other when in flight, he or she will rotate forward about the TAG and may land awkwardly on the front of the body; see Figure 3.73. This is what happens to many schoolchildren in the early stages of learning

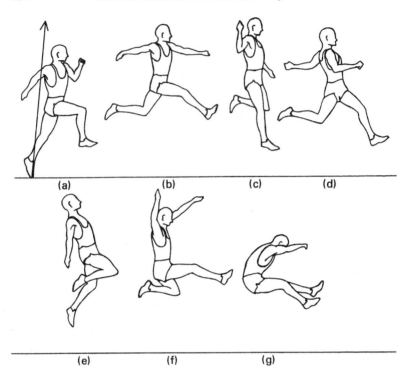

(a)   (b)   (c)   (d)

(e)   (f)   (g)

Figure 3.72

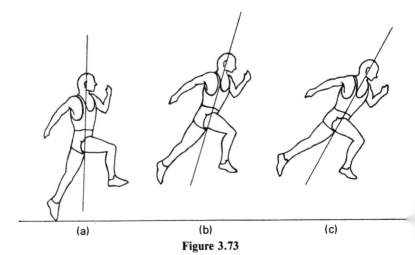

(a)   (b)   (c)

Figure 3.73

to long jump. In order to arrest the embarrassing forward rotation of the trunk, angular momentum can be transferred from the trunk to the arms and legs by increasing the angular velocity of the arms and legs relative to the TAG, i.e. if the arms are rotated cyclically about the transverse axis through the shoulder joints (TAS) and the legs are rotated in a similar way about the transverse axis through the hip joints (TAH), the angular momentum of the arms and legs about the TAG will be increased at the expense of the trunk, the angular velocity relative to the TAG and angular momentum about the TAG of which will decrease. If the rotation of the arms and legs about their respective local axes (TAS and TAH, respectively) is sufficiently vigorous, the angular velocity of the trunk may be reduced to zero or the direction of rotation may even be reversed; see Figure 3.72(d) and (e). The hitch-kick technique, therefore, enables the jumper to make full use of the ground reaction force at take-off in generating maximum upward velocity of the c. of g. and also to make a good landing on the feet.

In the piked dive and the hitch-kick technique of long jumping angular momentum of the whole body about the TAG is generated during the take-off period by an eccentric ground reaction force. The angular momentum is then transferred to and from various parts of the body. In some other activities, angular momentum is first of all generated in one or more body parts and then transferred to the rest of the body. For example, consider Figure 3.74 which shows a sequence of drawings taken from 12 frames of a film of a gymnast performing a standing back somersault. The frame speed of the film was 64 frames per second. Prior to take-off the arms are 'wound up' by swinging them anticlockwise (in Figure 3.74) about a transverse axis through the shoulder joints (TAS) to a position of full shoulder extension; see position 1. At this stage, the body has no angular momentum about any axis. From position 1 the arms are swung very rapidly about the TAS in a clockwise direction. At take-off the arms are moving very rapidly and have considerable angular momentum about the TAS; see position 11. After leaving the floor, any rotation of the whole body in the median plane will take place about a transverse axis through the whole-body c. of g. (TAG). Just after take-off, the arms have a certain backward angular momentum about the TAG since they are rotating very rapidly backwards with respect to this axis. A decrease in the angular velocity of the arms relative to the TAG will result in a decrease in the angular momentum of the arms about the TAG. Since the angular momentum of the whole body about the TAG is conserved during the flight phase, a decrease in the angular momentum of the arms will result in an increase in the angular momentum of the rest of the body. Just after take-off the angular velocity of the arms relative to the TAG is very rapidly reduced to zero. The loss in backward

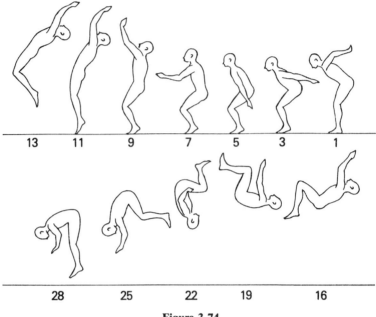

Figure 3.74

angular momentum thus incurred by the arms is simultaneously gained by the rest of the body and helps to rotate the whole body backwards about the TAG. During the time period between positions 11 and 22, over half the flight time, the angular velocity of the arms relative to the TAG is not only reduced to zero but the direction of rotation of the arms is reversed (anticlockwise in Figure 3.74) thereby increasing the backward angular momentum of the rest of the body even more. Evidently the greater the backward angular velocity of the arms at take-off, the greater will be their angular momentum about the TAG, and consequently the greater the amount of angular momentum which can be transferred to the rest of the body. One of the major faults made by individuals when learning the standing back somersault is the tendency to reduce the angular velocity of the arms just prior to take-off. For maximum benefit to be gained from the arms, the performer must continue to accelerate the arms until just *after* take-off.

Although the transfer of angular momentum from the arms to the rest of the body is an essential feature of the technique of performing a standing back somersault, the backward angular momentum generated in the arms prior to take-off is not usually the entire source of backward angular momentum of the whole body. If, as usually

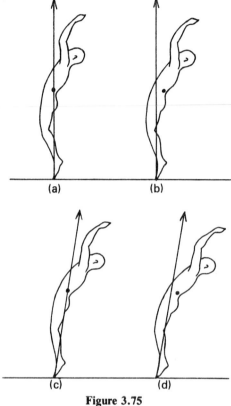

Figure 3.75

happens, the line of action of the ground reaction passes in front of the whole-body c. of g. just prior to take-off, a certain amount of backward angular momentum of the whole body, in addition to that possessed by the arms, will thus be obtained. Figure 3.75 shows four possible lines of action of the ground reaction in relation to the whole-body c. of g. at take-off. Assume that the speed of arm movement is the same in each case. In Figure 3.75(a) the ground reaction is vertical and passes directly through the whole-body c. of g. Therefore, the total backward angular momentum of the whole body just after take-off is that possessed by the arms. In Figure 3.75(b) the ground reaction is still vertical but the line of action of the ground reaction is in front of the whole-body c. of g. Consequently, the total backward angular momentum of the whole body just after take-off is the sum of that possessed by the arms and that resulting from the eccentric ground reaction force just prior to take-off. Clearly, the additional angular momentum afforded by the eccentric ground reaction should enable the performer to complete the somersault more easily than if he or she has to rely entirely on the angular momentum generated in the arms alone. In both cases, the ground reaction prior to take-off is vertical and, therefore, the whole-body c. of g. will move up and down vertically during the performance of the somersault; the c. of g. will not 'travel' horizontally. The feet would land on the same spot from which they took off if the orientation of the body parts to each other was the same at take-off and landing. In Figure 3.75(c) the line of action of the ground reaction passes through the whole-body c. of g. but is inclined with respect to the vertical. Therefore, the ground reaction has a horizontal as well as a vertical component. The rotary effects of the components, i.e. the turning moments exerted on the body about the transverse axis through the c. of g., cancel each other out. The linear effect of the vertical component is to lift the c. of g. vertically and the linear effect of the horizontal component is to push the c. of g. horizontally backwards; the c. of g. 'travels' horizontally during the performance of the somersault. In Figure 3.75(d), the line of action of the ground reaction is inclined at an angle to the vertical and passes in front of the c. of g. The linear effects of the two components will be similar to those in the situation depicted in Figure 3.75(c) but the rotary effect of the vertical component will be greater than that of the horizontal component, thereby generating backward angular momentum of the whole body about the transverse axis through the c. of g.

3.15 Rotation and Newton's Third Law of Motion

From Newton's First Law of Motion, the angular momentum of an object about a particular axis can only be changed by the action of an external turning moment. Internal forces can alter the moment of inertia of the object about its axis of rotation but provided it is not acted on by any external forces, the angular momentum of the object will be conserved. When internal forces alter the moment of inertia of an object about a particular axis, there is a simultaneous change in the angular momentum of each individual part of the object. For example, consider once again Figure 3.71 which shows four successive positions of a diver performing a forward piked dive. The pike is achieved by flexing the hips which simultaneously increases the angular momentum of the upper body and decreases the angular momentum of the legs about the transverse axis through the whole-body c. of g. (TAG), so that the angular momentum of the whole body about the TAG is conserved. When the hip flexor muscles contract to produce the piked position, they pull equally on both of their attachments, the upper body and the legs. Therefore, the impulse of the hip flexor turning moment on the upper body is exactly the same in magnitude but opposite in direction to that exerted on the legs, so that the angular momentum of the body about the local transverse axis through the hip joints (TAH) is unchanged; it remains at zero. To straighten out his or her body in preparation for entry into the water, the diver contracts the hip extensor muscles, which pull equally on both of their attachments – the upper body and legs. The impulse of the hip extensor turning moment on the upper body is equal in magnitude but opposite in direction to that exerted on the legs so that the angular momentum of the body about the TAH remains unchanged at zero. However, the action of the hip extensors also results in an increase in the angular momentum of the legs about the TAG and a decrease in the angular momentum of the upper body about the TAG so that the angular momentum of the whole body about the TAG is conserved. From the above discussion it follows that when an object is rotating about a particular axis with constant angular momentum such as the human body about the TAG during the flight phase of a jump, dive or somersault, the angular momentum of the body about any local axis will be zero.

In the piked dive, the actions of the hip flexors in piking the body and the hip extensors in straightening the body by rotating the upper body and legs in opposite directions are examples of the operation of Newton's Third Law of Motion as it applies to rotation. The law may be expressed as follows;

> *When an object A exerts a turning moment on another*
> *object B, there will be an equal and opposite turning*
> *moment exerted by object B on object A.*

The law may be demonstrated by using a turntable which is free to rotate about a vertical axis through its point of support. A man stands on the turntable, perfectly still with his arms outstretched at his sides; see overhead view in Figure 3.76(a). If the man flexes his left shoulder joint such that his left arm is rotated with respect to the rest of the

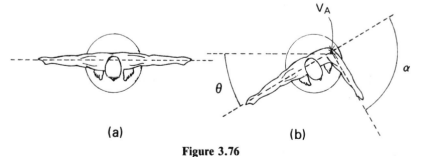

(a)   (b)

Figure 3.76

system (man and turntable) through an angle α in a horizontal plane about the local vertical axis V_A through his left shoulder joint, the rest of the sytem will be seen to rotate about V_A in the opposite direction to that of the arm through an angle θ; see Figure 3.76(b). Since the impulse of the shoulder flexor turning moment on the left arm is equal in magnitude but opposite in direction to that exerted on the rest of the system, the angular momentum of the whole system about V_A remains unchanged, i.e. zero. In Figure 3.76(b),

$$I_A\omega_A \text{ (clockwise)} = I_R\omega_R \text{ (anticlockwise)}$$

where

I_A = moment of inertia of the left arm about V_A

I_R = moment of inertia of the rest of the system about V_A

ω_A = angular velocity of the left arm about V_A

ω_R = angular velocity of the rest of the system about V_A

Since

$$\omega_A = \frac{\alpha}{t} \quad \text{and} \quad \omega_R = \frac{\theta}{t}$$

where t = time of application of shoulder flexor turning moment, then

$$I_A\alpha = I_R\theta$$

Therefore,

$$\theta = \frac{I_A\alpha}{I_R}$$

If, for example, $I_A/I_R = 1/3$, and $\alpha = 90°$, then $\theta = 30°$. The reaction of the rest of the human body to rotation of one part of the body is not always discernible especially when the larger part is in contact with the floor. In such cases, the reaction of the larger part may be prevented from occurring by friction between the larger part and the floor. The effect of Newton's third law is most clearly seen in movements which occur during flight when the body has no angular momentum; for example, a pike jump as shown in Figure 3.77(a) and (b), and the spiking action in volleyball as shown in Figure 3.77(c) and (d).

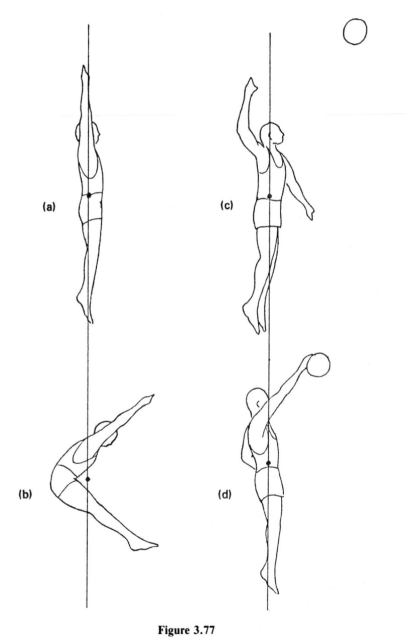

Figure 3.77

Appendix

Table 1 The English system of units

Measure	1	2
Distance	foot (ft)	foot (ft)
Speed	foot per second (ft/sec)	foot per second (ft/sec)
Acceleration	foot per second per second (ft/sec^2)	foot per second per second (ft/sec^2)
Mass	pound (lb)	slug
Linear momentum	pound foot per second (lb ft/sec)	slug foot per second (slug ft/sec)
Force	poundal (pdl) $1\,\text{pdl} = 1\,\text{lb} \times 1\,\text{ft/sec}^2$	pound force (lb f) $1\,\text{lb f} = 1\,\text{slug} \times 1\,\text{ft/sec}^2$
Weight	pound weight (lb wt) $1\,\text{lb wt} = 32.2\,\text{pdl}$	slug weight (slug wt) $1\,\text{slug wt} = 32.2\,\text{lb f}$
Angular distance	radian (rad)	radian (rad)
Angular speed	radian per second (rad/sec)	radian per second (rad/sec)
Angular acceleration	radian per second per second (rad/sec^2)	radian per second per second (rad/sec^2)
Moment of inertia	pound foot squared (lb ft^2)	slug foot squared (slug ft^2)
Angular momentum	pound foot squared per sec $(\text{lb ft}^2/\text{sec})$	slug foot squared per sec $(\text{slug ft}^2/\text{sec})$
Turning moment	poundal foot (pdl ft)	pound force foot (lb f ft)

Table 2 The metric system of units

Measure	1	2
Distance	centimetre (cm)	metre (m)
Speed	centimetre per second (cm/s)	metre per second (m/s)
Acceleration	centimetre per second per second (cm/s^2)	metre per second per second (m/s^2)
Mass	gram (g)	kilogram (kg)
Linear momentum	gram centimetre per second (g cm/s)	kilogram metre per second (kg m/s)
Force	dyne (dyn) $1 \, dyn = 1 \, g \times 1 \, cm/s^2$	newton (N) $1 \, N = 1 \, kg \times 1 \, m/s^2$
Weight	gram weight (g wt) $1 \, g \, wt = 981 \, dyn$	kilogram weight (kg wt) $1 \, kg \, wt = 9.81 \, N$
Angular distance	radian (rad)	radian (rad)
Angular speed	radian per second (rad/s)	radian per second (rad/s)
Angular acceleration	radian per second per second (rad/s^2)	radian per second per second (rad/s^2)
Moment of inertia	gram centimetre squared (g cm^2)	kilogram metre squared (kg m^2)
Angular momentum	gram centimetre squared per second (g cm^2/s)	kilogram metre squared per second (kg m^2/s)
Turning moment	dyne centimetre (dyn cm)	newton metre (N m)

Index